IMMEDIATE LIFE SUPPORT
FOR HEALTHCARE PRACTITIONERS

A STEP-BY-STEP GUIDE

BLESSING ISAACKSON

DISCLAIMER

The materials presented in this book are presented for information only and may be subject to change. Healthcare professionals should always follow their own local procedures and guidelines set by their regulatory bodies and must stick to their limitations.

Table of Contents

FORWARD

Fairview Training is committed to providing excellent learning resources to our learners to assist them in achieving their CPD requirements.

This step-by-step guide has been written to assist healthcare professionals to bolster their CPR skills and should form an integral resource in their face–to–face classroom training.

Learners can use this material during the training as a reference even when they have completed the course.

Blessing Isaackson

Managing Director,

Fairview Training Ltd

AIMS OF PROVIDING BASIC LIFE SUPPORT

Preserve the patient's life.

Prevent their condition from getting worse.

Promote the recovery of the patient.

MINIMISE THE RISK OF INFECTION.

Wear physical barriers such as Gloves, an Apron, a face shield, and a face mask to minimize the risk of infection.

ALERTING THE EMERGENCY MEDICAL SERVICES

Call 999 or 112 as a matter of urgency.

A lone helper with a mobile phone must call 999 or 112 and then start CPR immediately if the patient is unresponsive and not breathing.

A lone helper without a mobile phone should go for help and then commence CPR.

Within a hospital environment, the number to call is 2222.

PRIMARY SURVEY

This is the initial assessment conducted to determine if there are any life-threatening issues facing the patient that need to be addressed in order of priority.

Assess the environment for danger- make sure you and the patient are safe.

Check the patient's response by giving verbal commands to the patient. For example, "Open your eyes" or "Squeeze my hand".

Ensure the patient's airway is patent- by conducting a head tilt, and chin lift. Ensure the patient is breathing normally- look out for agonal gasping.

D-Danger

R -Response

A-Airway

B-Breathing

C-Circulation

DO NOT ATTEMPT RESUSCITATION

Always communicate with the patient and seek their consent before treatment unless the patient is unresponsive in which case you are assumed to have their implied permission.

A patient may withdraw their consent to CPR and this is only related to CPR if they sign up for a Do not attempt CPR. (DNAR). You must respect the DNAR.

Chain of survival

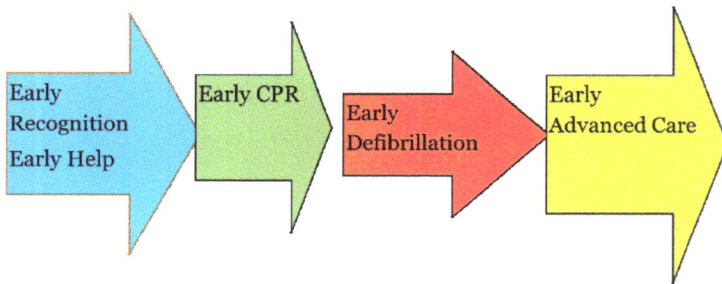

Calling for Help

Call 999 or 112 and give them the following information:

Your location

The help you require.

Name of patient

Number of patients

THE STRUCTURE OF THE HEART

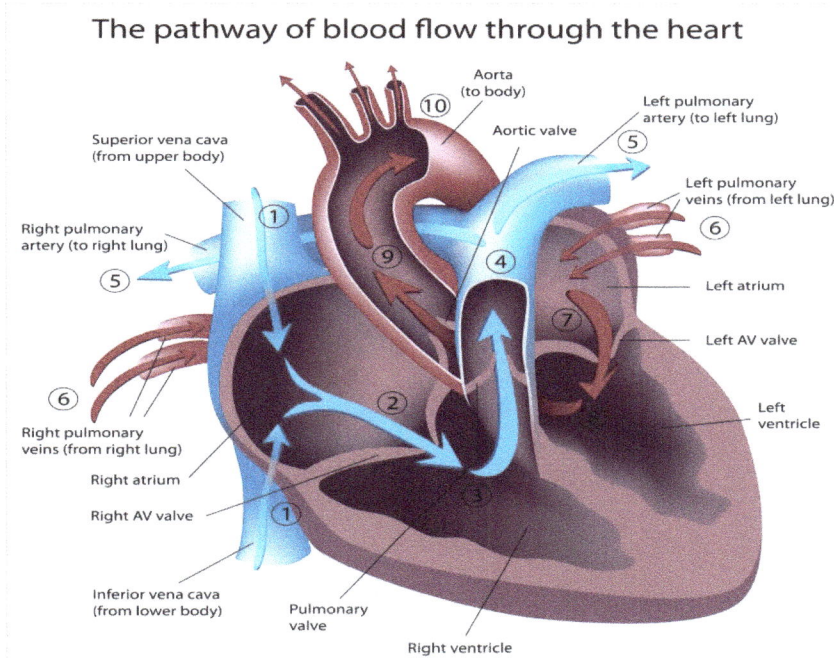

The pathway of blood flow through the heart

The heart comprises an upper chamber and a lower chamber. The upper chambers are made up of the left atrium and the right atrium and the lower chambers are made up of the left ventricle and the right ventricle. The heart also comprises the septum, which is the wall of tissue separating the left and the sides of the heart. The septum is made up of the atrial and ventricular septums.

The functions of the Left and right sides of the heart

Right Side- Receives de-oxygenated blood that has traversed the whole of the body and sends it to the heart to receive fresh oxygenated blood and circulates the freshly oxygenated blood to the rest of the body.

Left Side- The left side receives the freshly oxygenated blood and circulates it to the whole of the body.

The role of arteries, veins, and capillaries

Arteries- Carry oxygenated blood from the rest of the heart to the rest of the body. The coronary arteries supply blood to the heart muscle. They can be found on the outer part of the heart.

Veins- carry de-oxygenated blood from the rest of the body back to the heart.

Capillaries- these are a network of smaller blood vessels that connect the arteries and veins.

THE VALVES IN THE HEART

TYPES OF VALVES IN THE HEART-

On the right side of the heart-

Tricuspid valve- allows blood flow from the right atrium to the right ventricle.

Pulmonary valve- controls the flow of oxygen-poor blood from the heart to the lungs.

Each time the heart beats the valves open and close enabling a one-directional flow of blood.

Left Side of the heart

Mitral valve- located between the left atrium and the left ventricle.

Aortic valve- controls blood from the left ventricle to the aorta

THE HEART on the left ventricle

- The heart's electrical system sends signals that dictate when the heart contracts and relaxes to send blood pumping around the body.

- The signals are dispatched by the sinus node which is the heart's pacemaker.

THREE LAYERS OF THE HEART MUSCLE

THE PERICADIUM-the thin outer layer of the heart

THE MYOCARDIUM- This is a muscular middle layer of the heart. This part contracts and relaxes to pump blood around the heart.

THE ENDOCARDIUM– this is a thin inner layer of the heart. It forms the lining of all the chambers of the heart including the valves.

SEPTUM- this separates the left and the right side of the heart. It ensures the oxygenated blood never mixes with the deoxygenated blood.

HOW OXYGEN GETS TO THE BLOOD

OXYGEN GETS TO THE BLOOD IN 4 WAYS

THE RIGHT ATRIUM- receives blood with a low level of oxygen from the rest of the body. It then pumps the blood down the **right ventricle.**

RIGHT VENTRICLE- pumps the blood to the lungs to get oxygenated.

LEFT ATRIUM- Receives the highly oxygenated blood from the lungs and pumps it to the left ventricle.

 LEFT VENTRICLE – the left ventricle then pumps the blood to the rest of the body.

THE HEART'S CONDUCTION SYSTEM

The heart's conduction system is a network of nodes, cells, and electrical signals that keep the heart beating.

- Sinoatrial Node (SA node)-
- Atrioventricular node-
- Bundle of His (Atrioventricular bundle)-
- Punkinje fibres-

SINOATRIAL NODE

This is the heart's natural pacemaker. It sends electrical signals which starts the heartbeat. It is in the upper part of the heart's right atrium. How fast or slow the SA nodes send electrical signals depends on the autonomic nervous system, which includes the sympathetic nervous system and the parasympathetic nervous system.

The sympathetic nervous system makes the sinoatrial node work faster, making the heart beat faster.

The **parasympathetic node** makes the SA node work slower and, therefore, a slower heartbeat.

ATRIOVENTRICULAR NODE (AV NODE)

The AV Node controls the heart's rate. It generates impulses for the heart's contraction and coordinates the blood flow between the upper and lower chambers of the heart. The electrical impulses generated by the AV node help the heart contract and pump blood. It acts as a gatekeeper to briefly delay the impulses from the SA node. That delay allows the full contraction of the atria, enabling blood to be fully emptied from the atria to the ventricles.

BUNDLE OF HIS

The bundle of HIS is also known as the atrioventricular bundle. It is located between the atrium and the ventricles of the heart. The

Bundle of HIS helps to transmit the electrical impulse from the AV node to the Purkinje Fibres.

PUNKINJE FIBRES

These are specialized ventricular fibres found in the inner ventricular walls of the heart. They assist in the contraction of the ventricles and in maintaining the rhythm of the heart.

HEART ATTACK

Heart attack results from the death of parts of the cardiac muscles caused by blockage in the coronary artery from cholesterol plaque, thrombus, or spasm. Heart attack may also be called Myocardial infarction. When there is a blood clot in the coronary artery, the area beyond the blockage does not receive blood and that can lead to depletion of oxygen and other nutrients which the heart muscles rely on to survive leading to a heart attack.

RECOGNISING HEART ATTACK

Excruciating pain in the centre of the chest can spread to one or both arms, the jaw back, and shoulders. Pain associated with a heart attack is not relieved by resting.

The patient is breathless.

A general feeling of indigestion.

Faintness and dizziness.

The patient will be anxious and have a feeling of impending doom.

They become cyanotic. The pulse is rapid and gradually becomes weak and irregular.

Sweating is also associated with patients experiencing a heart attack.

They are often gasping for air.

MANAGING HEART ATTACK

STEP 1

Call 999/112 and inform the handler that you suspect a heart attack.

STEP 2

Place the patient in a comfortable position preferably in a half-sitting position to reduce the stress on the heart. The head and shoulders should be supported, and the knees bent. Place a cushion or pillow at the back to support them.

STEP 3

If available, give 300 mg of aspirin to the patient. The aspirin can be dissolved in water, or it can be given to the patient to chew.

STEP 4

If they have angina medication such as GTN spray or tablet, help them to take it.

STEP 5

Only provide oxygen to patient's experiencing a heart attack if they are hypoxaemic[1]. In a hypoxaemic patient adjust the oxygen flow and

---

[1] NICE. Chest Pain - Scenario: Management. 2020. Available at https://cks.nice.org.uk/chest-pain#!scenario (accessed April 2020).

titrate the patient's oxygen saturation levels to between 94-98% SPO2 and for a COPD patient titrate the oxygen levels to 88-92% SPO2.

STEP 6

Continue to monitor their vital signs before help arrives.

APSPIRIN

It is an antiplatelet which stops platelets from sticking together. It is a pain reliever, reduces inflammation, and prevents or reduces fever. It prevents the blood clot from getting larger.

Classification-

ACTION

This medication helps to reduce blood clot formation.

CONTRA—INDICATIONS

CONTRA-INDICATIONS FOR ASPIRIN

Active peptic ulceration, bleeding disorders, children under the age of 16 years (due to the risk of Reye's syndrome) unless specifically indicated, eg Kawasaki disease, which affects children under the age of 5 years. It is characterised by rash, swollen glands, cracked lips, swollen and red hands, and feet. Reyes's syndrome is a condition that affects children after they have had the flu and it can affect the brain if not treated speedily, Haemophilia, patients with a history of anaphylactic shock to aspirin, chronically asthmatic patients. Avoid giving it to patients taking certain anticoagulants such as heparin or warfarin.

PRESENTATION

Three hundred milligrams in tablet form. Patients should chew the tablet or have it dissolved in water.

CAUTIONS

In some patients, the benefits of administering aspirin far outweigh the risks of taking it. In the case of the following patients, the medication should be given despite the risk:

A patient with asthma

A pregnant woman

A patient with renal failure

A patient with moderate hepatic disease without jaundice

Gastric or duodenal ulcer

A patient undergoing treatment with anticoagulants.

SIDE EFFECTS

Risk of gastric bleeding

Wheezing in some asthmatics

ACUTE CORONARY SYNDROMES

Heart attack accounts for 64,000 deaths yearly.[2] Acute coronary syndrome covers all the conditions where the heart muscle is deprived of oxygen- a condition known as Ischaemia. It can occur because of stable angina or myocardial infarction.

The pathway of blood flow through the heart

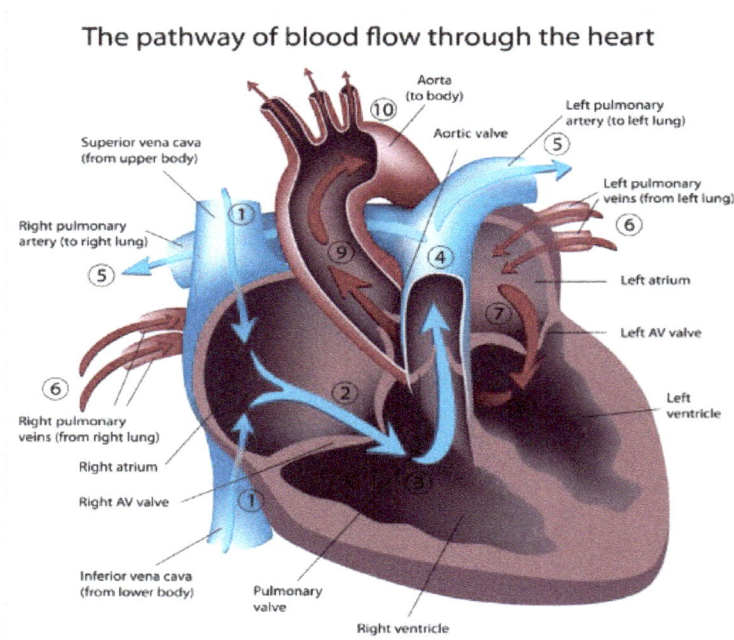

[2] Bhf.org.uk UK factsheet. Available from :https://www.bhf.org.uk/-
/media/files/research/heart-statistics/bhf-cvd-statistics-ukfactsheet.pdf?la=en.
Published MMARCH ")"!> Accessed June 6, 2022.

Stable Angina

This occurs when the heart does not receive the amount of oxygen that it requires. This can be alleviated by resting or providing oxygen to the patient. Stable angina occurs because of stress, physical exertion, or a change in the weather. Stable angina can be relieved by rest or medication.

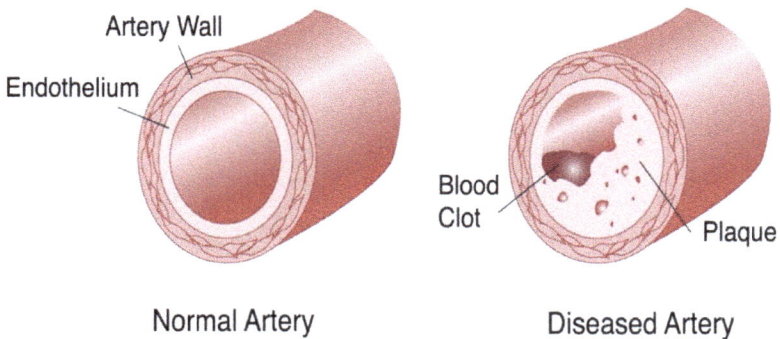

Normal Artery   Diseased Artery

Unstable angina

Unstable Angina occurs when there is a blood clot in the coronary arteries that is transient or occurs partially, leading to the symptoms of ischaemia, one of which is chest pain. This can happen even when the patient is at rest. Unstable angina may not be relieved by rest or by taking medication.

Signs and symptoms of Angina

- Chest pain triggered by physical exertion, change in the weather, and stress.
- Chest pain which subsides by the patient resting
- Pain in the centre of the chest which radiates to the jaw, back, shoulder, and back.
- Nausea or vomiting
- Breathlessness
- Dizziness
- Casualty is usually anxious.

Non-STEMI: If the unstable angina is not dealt with, this may lead to a non-STEMI. This is where the myocardium is affected by the ischaemia to the extent that the ST segment is not elevated on the ECG (Electrocardiogram).

Non-STEMI can be distinguished from unstable angina because of the increase in the production of cardiac enzymes emanating from the death of the cardiac tissue.

STEMI—ST segment elevation myocardial infarction—occurs when a blood clot completely blocks the coronary arteries, leading to permanent damage to the cardiac muscle cells. The difference between non-STEMI and STEMI on the ECG is that with STEMI, the ST segment is elevated on the ECG.

UNSTABLE ANGINA

MEDICATION	AGE OF PATIENT	ROUTE OF ADMINISTRATION	DOSAGE	DURATION
ASPIRIN DISPERSIBLE TABLETS	Adult	Mouth (chewable) Mouth (dispersed in water)	75Mg x 4 300Mg	
AND				
GLYCERYL TRINITRATE (AEROSOL SPRAY)	Adult	Sublingually	400 Micrograms	1-2 SPRAYS
OR				
GLYCERYL TRINTRATE	ADULT	TABLETS	300 Micrograms 400 micrograms 600 micrograms 0.3-1 mg	Repeat as required

GLYCERYL TRINITRATE

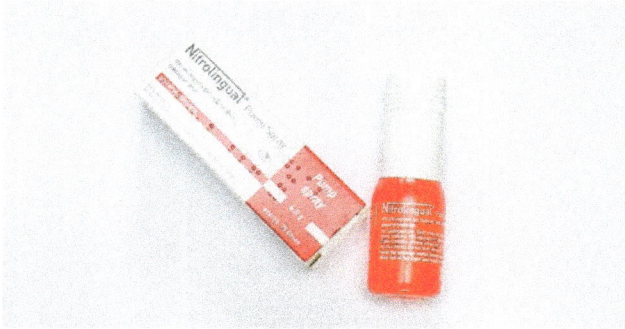

Non- STEMI- Non-ST Segment Elevation Myocardial Infarction

Treat like unstable angina

MEDICATION	AGE OF PATIENT	ROUTE OF ADMINISTRATION	DOSAGE	DURATION
ASPIRIN DISPERSIBLE TABLETS	Adult	Mouth (chewable) Mouth (dispersed in water)	75Mg x 4 300Mg	
AND				
GLYCERYL TRINITRATE (AEROSOL SPRAY)	Adult	Sublingually	400 Micrograms	every 5 minutes or as required

OR				
GLYCE RYL TRINT RATE	ADULT	TABLET S	300 Micrograms 400 micrograms 600 micrograms 0.3-1 mg	Repeat as required

ST SEGMENT ELEVATION MYOCARDIAL INFARCTION

MEDICATION	AGE OF PATIENT	ROUTE OF ADMINISTRATION	DOSAGE	DURATION
ASPIRIN DISPERSIBLE TABLETS	Adult	Mouth (chewable) Mouth (dispersed in water)	75Mg x 4 300Mg	
AND				
GLYCERYL TRINITRATE (AEROSOL SPRAY)	Adult	Sublingually	400 Micrograms	every 5 minutes or as required
OR				
GLYCERYL TRINTRATE	ADULT	TABLETS	300 Micrograms 400 micrograms 600 micrograms 0.3-1 mg	Repeat as required

GLYCERYL TRINTRATE (GTN) -

EMERGENCY MEDICATION FOR

RELIEVING ANGINA ATTACK

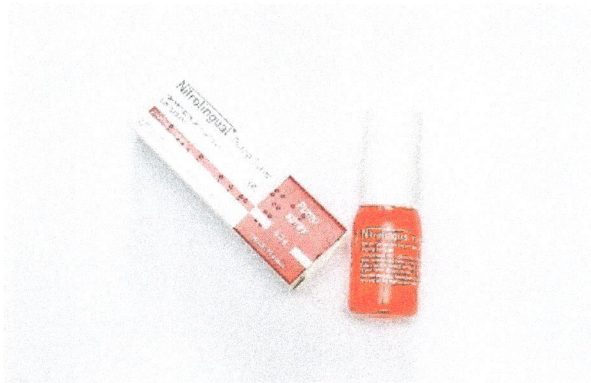

GTN can be administered in the form of a sublingual tablet or spray under the patient's mouth ensuring that the mouth is closed.

PRESENTATION

Spray –400 micrograms glyceryl trinitrate per metered dose.

Tablet– 300, 500, or 600 mcg per tablet.

INDICATIONS

To be administered when the patient is experiencing cardiac chest pain because of angina or myocardial infarction. The systolic blood pressure must be greater than 90mmHg.

To be administered to patients with suspected cocaine toxicity

ACTIONS

GTN is a vasodilator that helps to dilate the coronary arteries or relieve coronary spasms. It will also reduce the blood pressure.

CAUTIONS- make sure the nozzle of the spray does not contact the patient's mouth to avoid or minimise the risk of cross-contamination.

CONTRA-INDICATIONS

The medication should not be given where the patient is known to have:

Hypotension, head trauma, brain haemorrhage, or where the patient is known to have taken erectile dysfunction medications Viagra (Sildenafil) or Cialis (tadalafil) or vardenafil (Levitra) in the past 24 hours as this may lead to severe hypotension, hypovolaemia, unconscious patients.

SIDE EFFECTS

Headache, dizziness, and hypotension

ADMINSITRATION AND DOSAGE– one or two 400 micrograms metered doses.

DOSAGE AND ADMINISTRATION

Angina or myocardial infarction (systolic blood pressure is >90mm/Hg)

Adult

Sublingual tablet 1 tablet (0.3 to 0.4mg) every 5 minutes no maximum dose

Trans lingual Spray- (0.4mg) at 5 minutes interval- no maximum dose

Acute myocardial failure (systolic BP >110 mm/Hg)

Adult

Sublingual tablet- 1 tablet (0.3mg) at 5-minute intervals maximum of six tablets

Translingual spray- 1 spray (0.4mg) at 5-minute intervals- maximum six spray.

Administering GTN to a patient with left ventricular MI can lead to hypotension.

Normal Sinus Rhythm

This is a normal heart rhythm. A heart in a sinus Rhythm is beating between 60-100 beats in a minute. It is not a shockable rhythm.

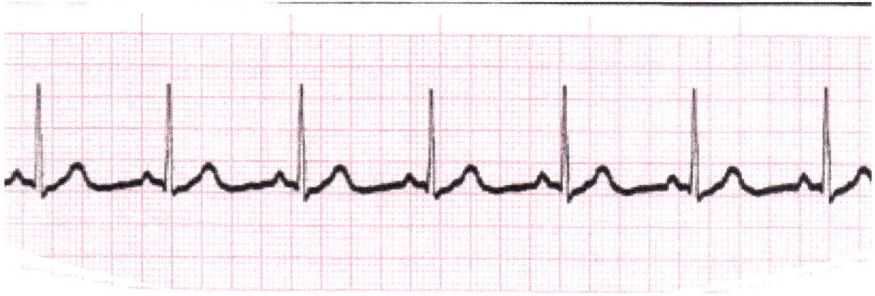

Heart Rhythms-Ventricular Fibrillation

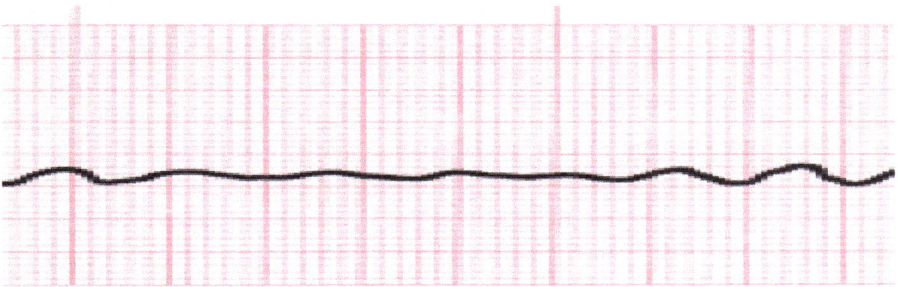

Pulseless Ventricular Tachycardia

It occurs when the heart rate exceeds 100 bpm.

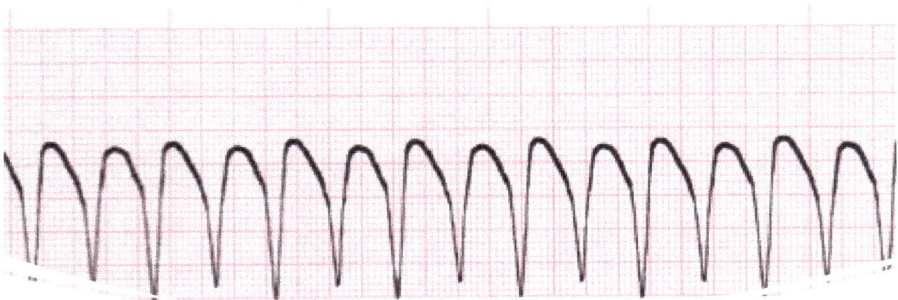

Asystole

The asystole rhythm occurs when there is a complete absence of electrical activity in the heart. A patient with this rhythm is clinically dead.

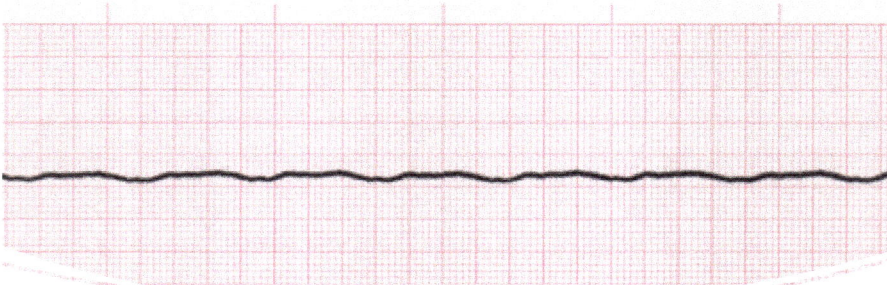

SUDDEN CARDIAC ARREST

- This happens when the heart stops suddenly.
- The survival rate is low about 10%.
- The rate of survival depends on factors of timing of CPR and the use of a defibrillator.

CAUSES OF CARDIAC ARREST

- **CAUSES**
- Myocardial infarction
- Pulmonary embolism
- Diabetic ketoacidosis
- Asthma.
- Sepsis
- Tension Pneumothorax
- Cardiac Tamponade
- Hypoxia
- Hypovolaemia
- Hypothermia
- Hypo/hyperkalaema.
- Toxins

Blood pressure

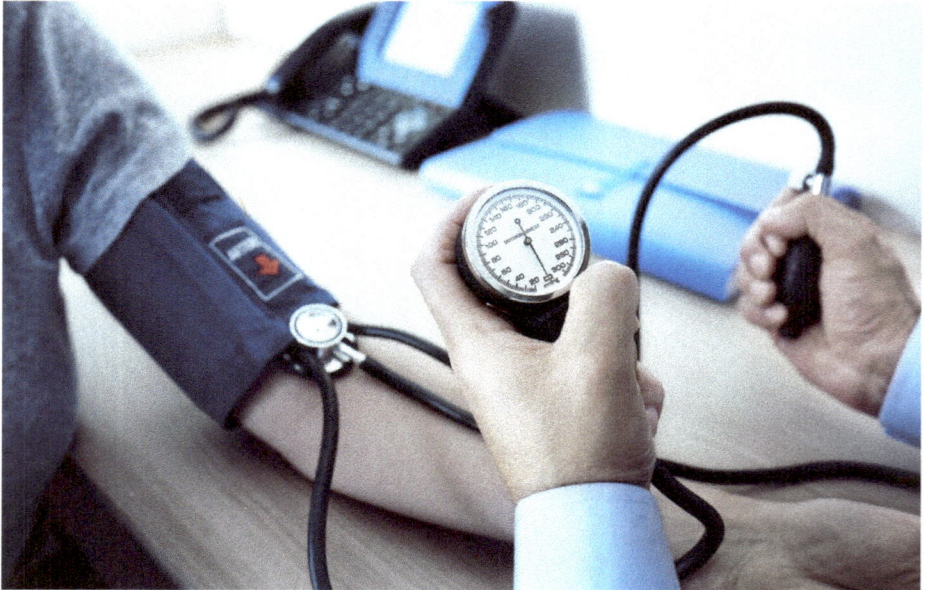

This is a measure of the pressure of the blood on the walls of the blood vessels.

The blood pressure record has two measurements:

Systolic blood Pressure is the BP when the ventricles contract and blood is forced from the heart. This is the higher reading of the BP.

Diastolic Blood Pressure is the BP when the ventricles relax. This is the lower reading of the blood pressure.

Blood pressure is measured in millimetres of mercury (mmHg). It is normally recorded as systolic over diastolic- 120/80.

Blood pressure values

Normal range

- Systolic -120-129 mmHg
- Diastolic-80-84 mmHg

Hypertension

Systolic 140 or higher

Diastolic-90 or higher

Hypotension

Systolic -90 mmHg or less

ADULT CPR

- If the patient becomes unresponsive, kneel beside him.
- Check if the casualty is responsive by shaking the shoulder, talking to the casualty, and giving commands "Wake up!" "Squeeze my hand."
- Place one hand on the forehead.
- Do a head tilt and chin lift. Place two fingers on the casualty's chin and one hand on the forehead and conduct a head tilt chin lift.
- Lower your head close to the casualty's face with your cheek close to the nose so that you can listen for any breath from the casualty's nose, feel the air from the casualty's nose on your cheek, and see the casualty's chest rise and fall. Do this for no more than 10 seconds.

- If the Casualty is not breathing, call 999/112 for emergency help and commence CPR.
- Place the heel of your hand in the centre of the patient's chest slightly above the tip of the breastbone. The position of your hand on the chest is vital to the performance of effective CPR.

AIRWAY MANAGEMENT

Manual Airway Manoeuvres

Head Tilt-Chin Lift

The head Tilt-chin lift should be done on a patient who has airway blockage resulting from loss of pharyngeal muscle tone. This manoeuvre should be averted if the patient is suspected to have a spinal injury.

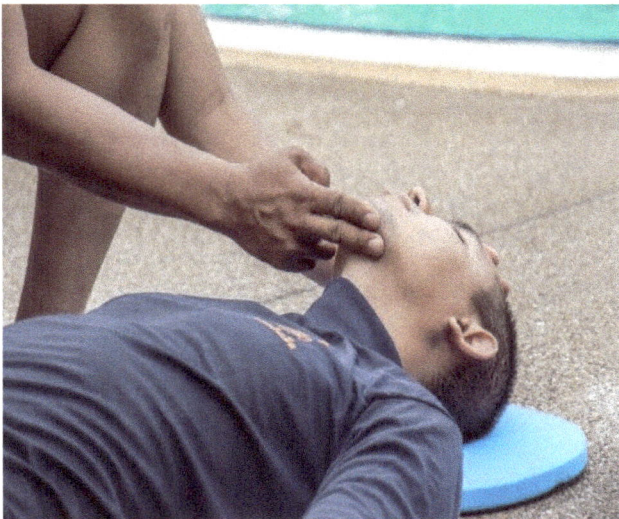

The advantages of using this technique are that its use does not involve any instrument and it is simple manoeuvre. Unfortunately, it does not protect the patient from the risk of aspiration and is contra-indicated for patients with spinal injury.

Jaw Thrust

The Jaw thrust should be done on a patient who has airway blockage resulting from loss of pharyngeal muscle tone. This manoeuvre should be averted if the patient is suspected to have a spinal injury.

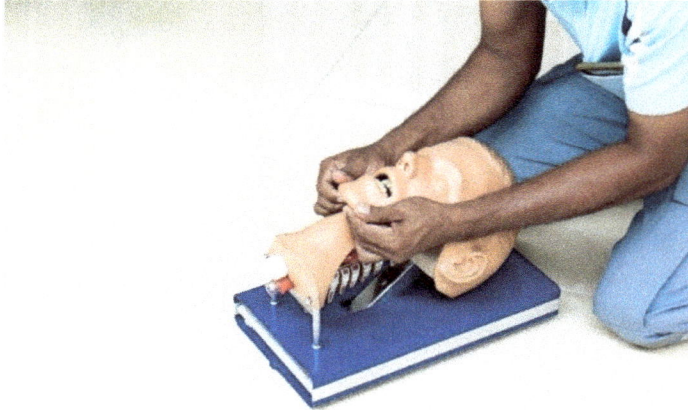

Suction

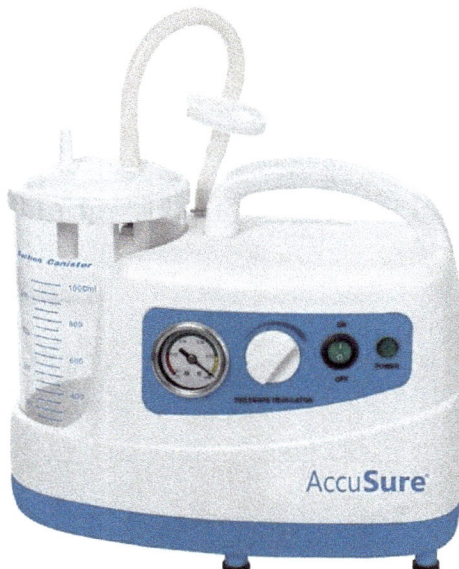

Whenever you can hear a gurgling sound, prepare to use suctions. The gurgling sound can be caused by blood, vomit, or secretions. Suctions assist in removing vomit and secretions. There are diverse types of suctions -mains operated, handheld, and reusable suctions.

Suctions are indicated for patients who cannot maintain or clear their own airway and prevent vomit or secretions from entering the lower respiratory tract and are contra-indicated for patients who can maintain or clear their own airway.

It prevents aspiration of vomit, blood, or secretions.

The disadvantage of the suction is that it not only removes fluid it also removes air thereby creating the risk of hypoxia. To avoid this, make sure the suctioning is short.

If all you are removing is a small amount of saliva you need a pressure of no more than 150 to 200 mmHg.[3]

---

[3] Randle J, Coffey F and Bradbury M, 2009. Oxford Handbook of Clinical Skills in Adult Nursing. Oxford: Oxford University Press.

AIRWAY ADJUNCTS

OROPHARYNGEAL AIRWAY

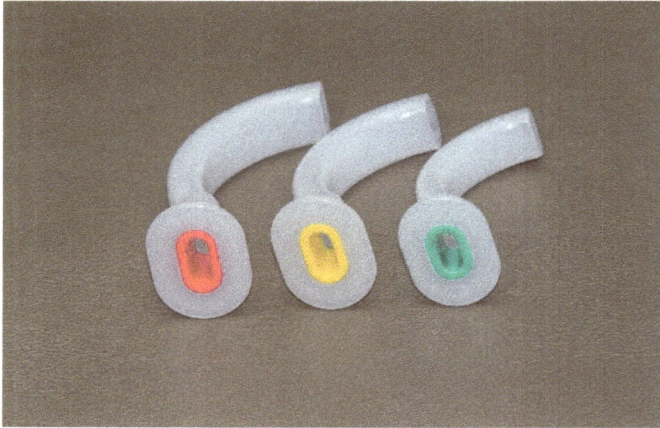

Step 1

Measure the OPA

Measure the distance between the patient's incisors and the angle of the jaw.

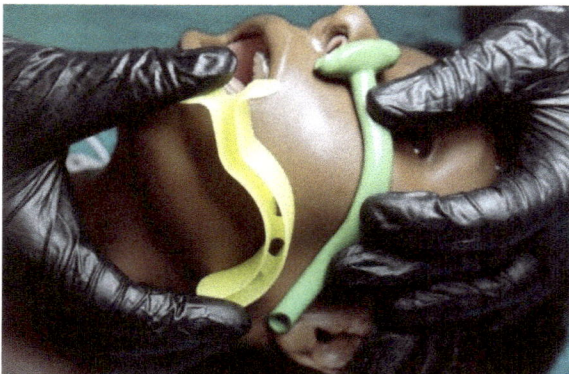

Step 2

Check the patient and clear any visible blood, vomit, or secretions with a suction if available.

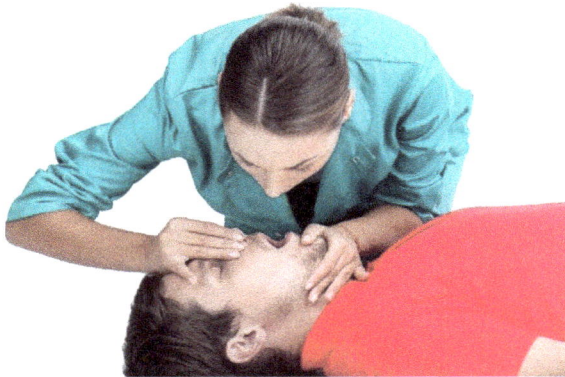

Step 3

Insert the OPA upside down so that the end touches the hard palate and glide along the hard palate until it touches the soft palate.

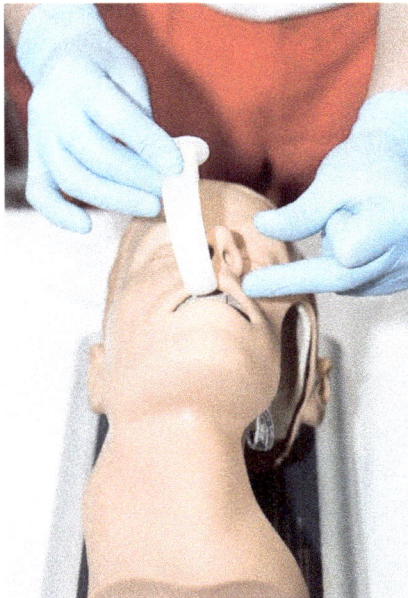

Step 4

Rotate the OPA 180°.

Step 5

Keep inserting the OPA until it gets to the pharynx and remove it if there is a sign of a gag reflex. If there is a gag reflex then revert to the head tilt and chin lift or the jaw thrust.

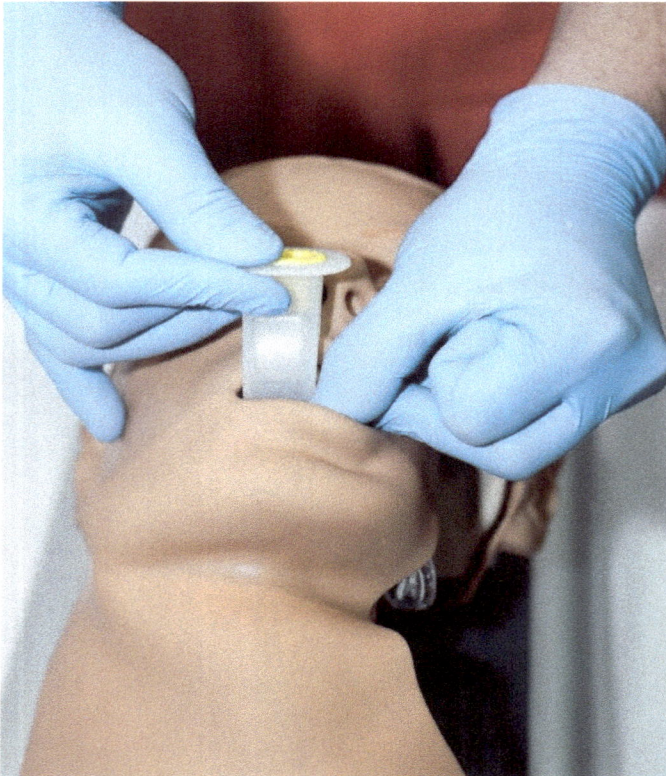

CHOKING

Choking occurs when there is a full or partial blockage of the airway. It occurs between the mouth and the carina– the part of the airway where the left and the right bronchi split from the bronchi.

Mild choking

This happens when the airway is partly blocked. With partial blockage, the patient still can speak. In this case, you should encourage him to cough, and they should be able to clear the obstruction themselves. If the obstruction does clear, then commence the back blows.

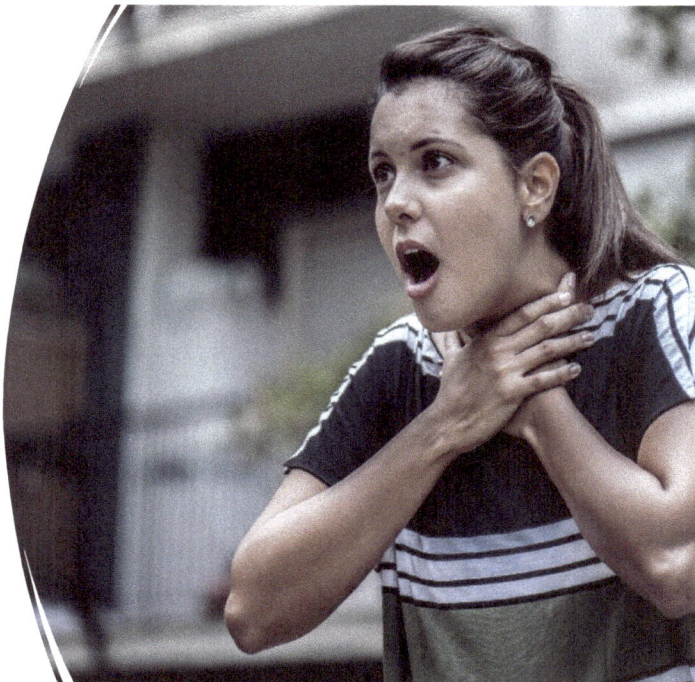

Severe Choking

Severe choking usually involves full blockage of the airway. The person will not be able to speak. To help them, you must immediately commence 5 back lows followed by 5 abdominal thrusts. If the treatment does not work the patient will at some point become unconscious and not breathing. You must commence CPR immediately.

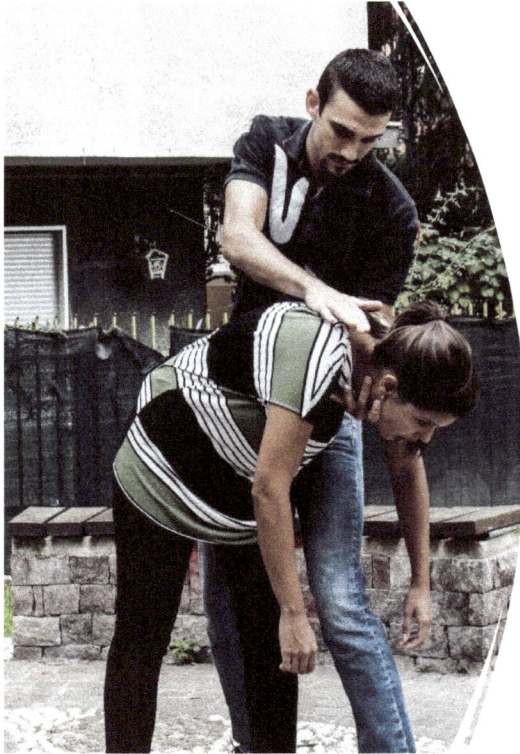

Abdominal thrusts

Make a fist with your dominant hand and then place that fist above the navel and below the tip of the sternum. Press backward and upwards up to 5 times.

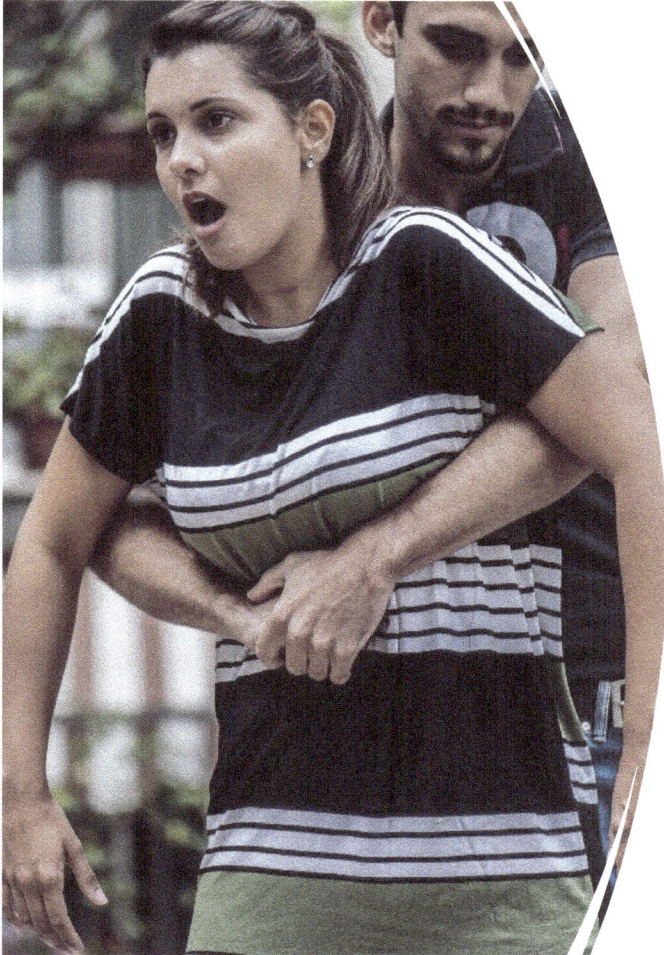

Choking Infant

No blind finger sweeps

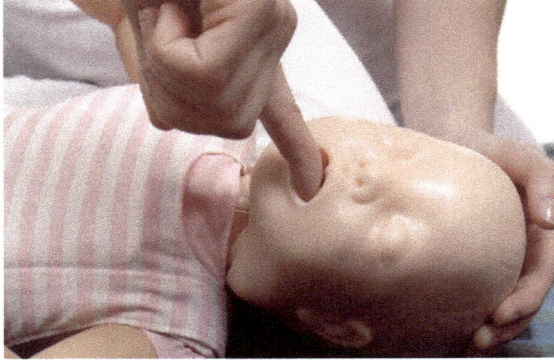

Choking Infant-Back blows.

Give up to five back blows with the heel of your hand. Adjust the blows to suit so they are commensurate with the size of the baby you are treating. The blows between the shoulder blades are necessary to remove the obstruction, but excessive back blows may cause severe damage to the baby.

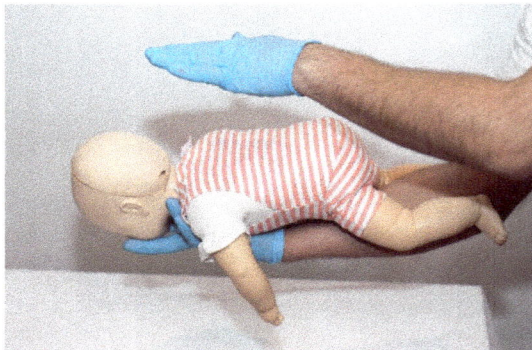

Choking Infant-Back blows.

Give up to five back blows using the heel of your hand and between the shoulder blades.

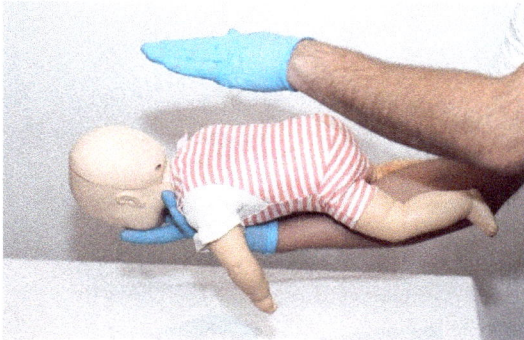

Choking Infant

Chest Thrust

Give up to five chest thrusts with two fingers in the centre of the infant's chest and then call for help if the chest thrusts have not worked to clear the obstructions.

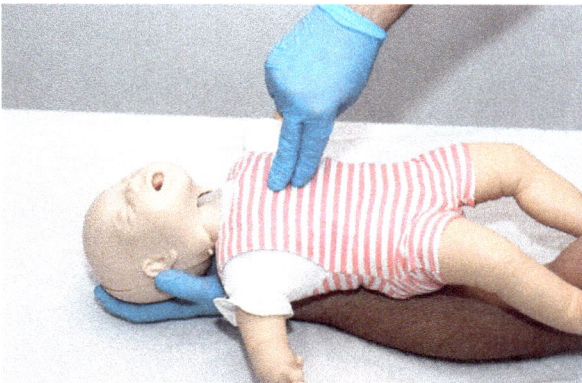

Choking Infant

When to call for help

After administering the five back blows and the five chest thrusts, if the treatment has not worked, it is vital that you call or get a colleague to call 999 or 112.

ADULT CPR

STEP 1

Kneel beside the patient.

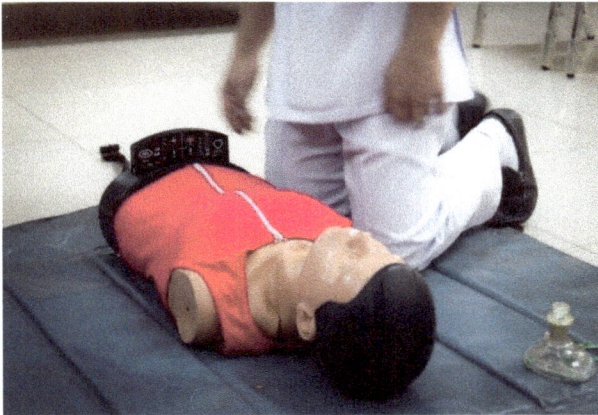

STEP 2

Check around for danger; Make sure the patient is safe and you are also safe!

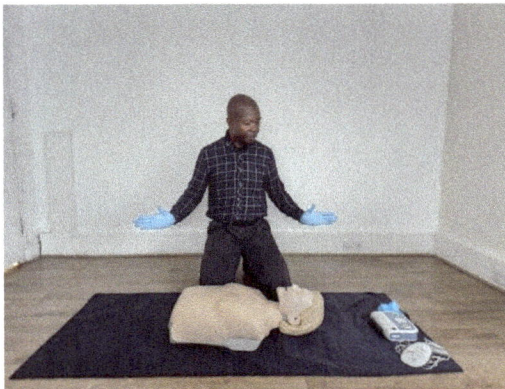

Step 3

Check if the patient is responsive.

Tap on the shoulder or squeeze on the patient's earlobes.

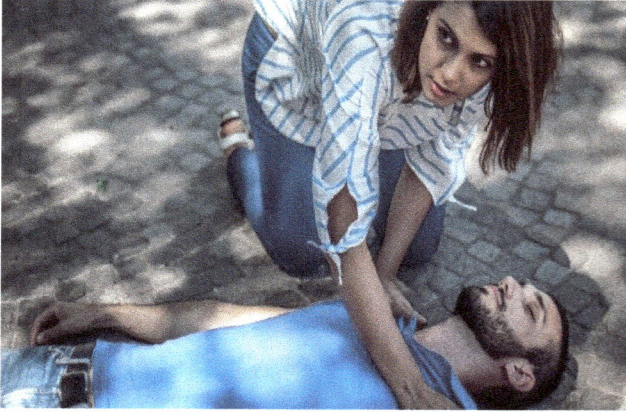

Step 4

Place one on the forehead.

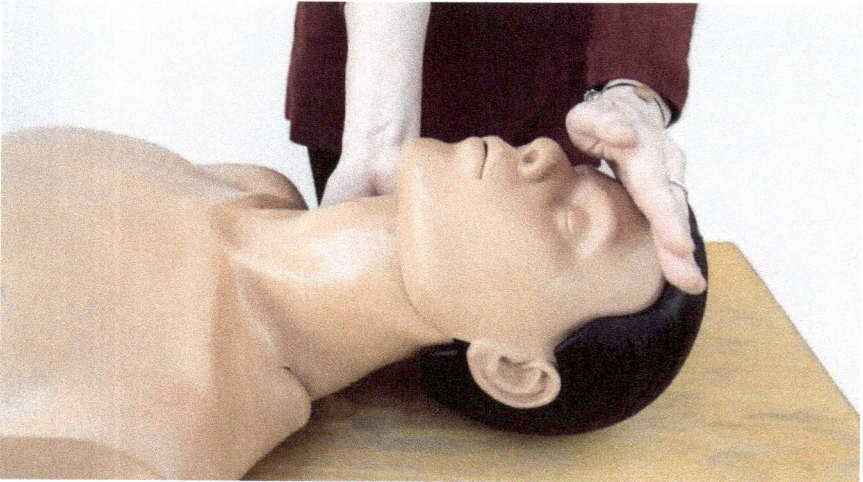

Step 5

Do a head tilt and a chin lift to maintain a clear airway.

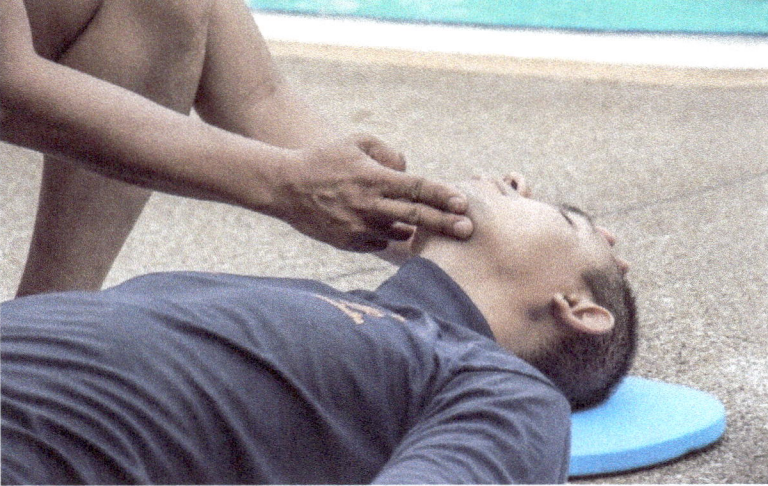

Step 6

Look, listen, and feel for breathing.

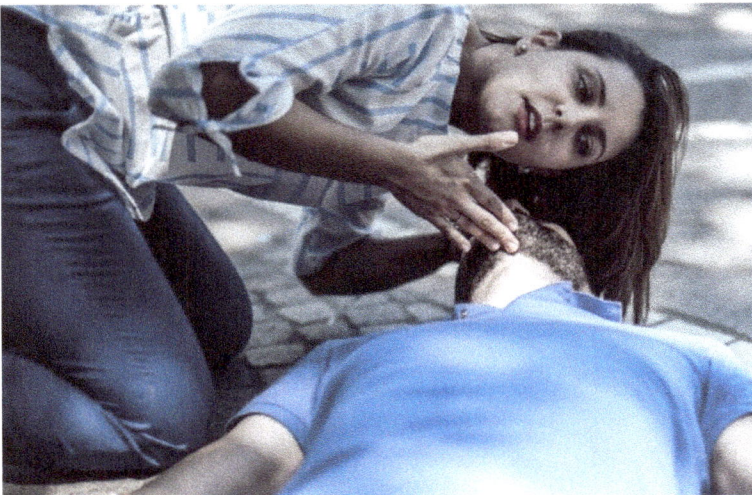

Step 7

Call 999/112

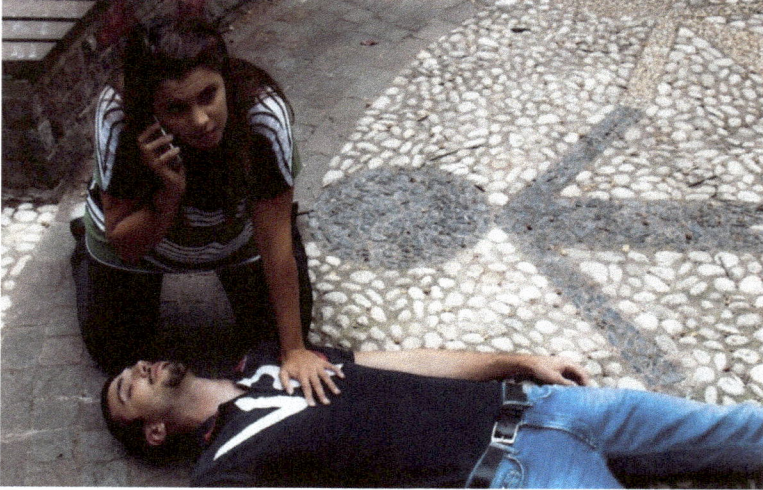

Step 8

Start chest compressions at a ratio of 30 chest compressions to 2 rescue breaths.

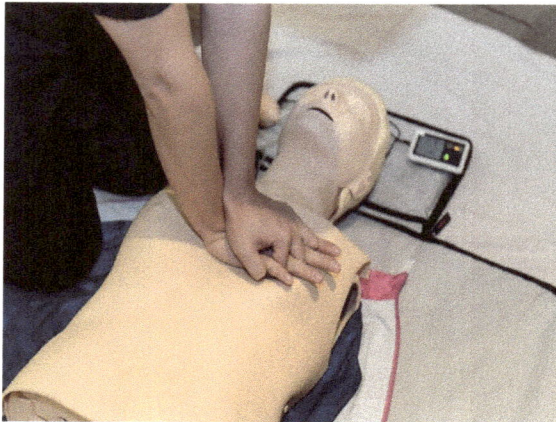

STEP 9

RESCUE BREATHS

Rescue breathing can be performed with a face mask over the face of the casualty as a barrier against infections. Squeeze the nose with your thumb and index finger with the patient's head tilted back to maintain an open airway.

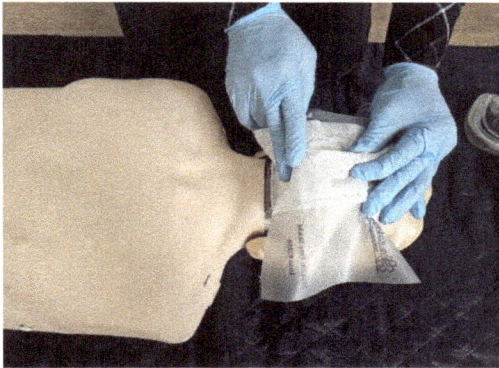

STEP 10

Seal your mouth over the patient's mouth and give two rescue breaths if it is safe to do so.

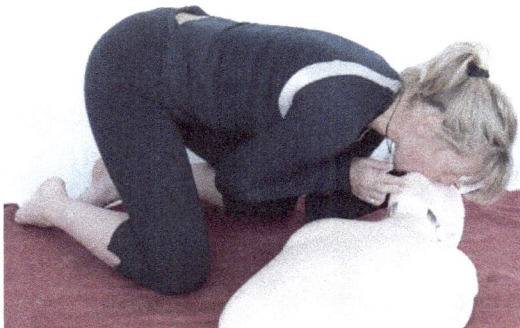

STEP 11

Seal your mouth over the patient's mouth.

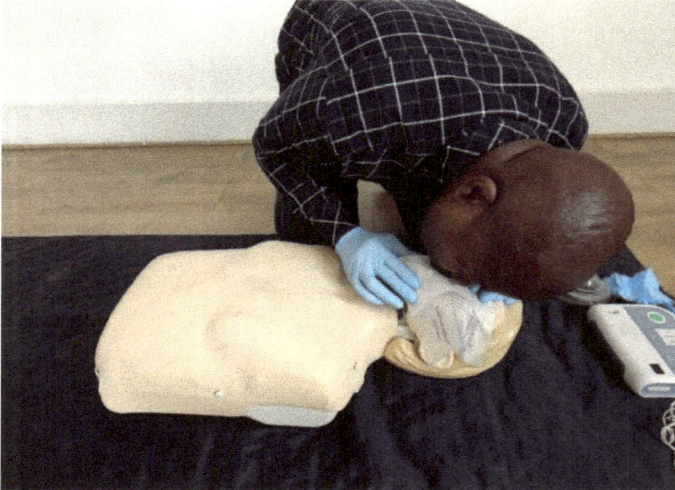

Or mouth-to-pocket mask

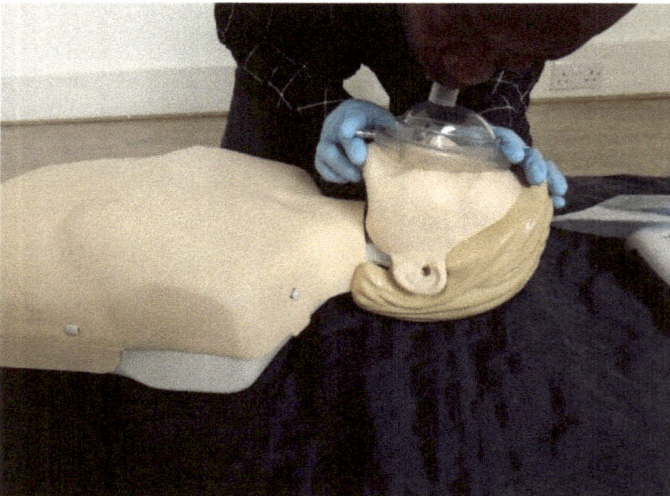

Mouth to a Bag Valve Mask, two-person technique.

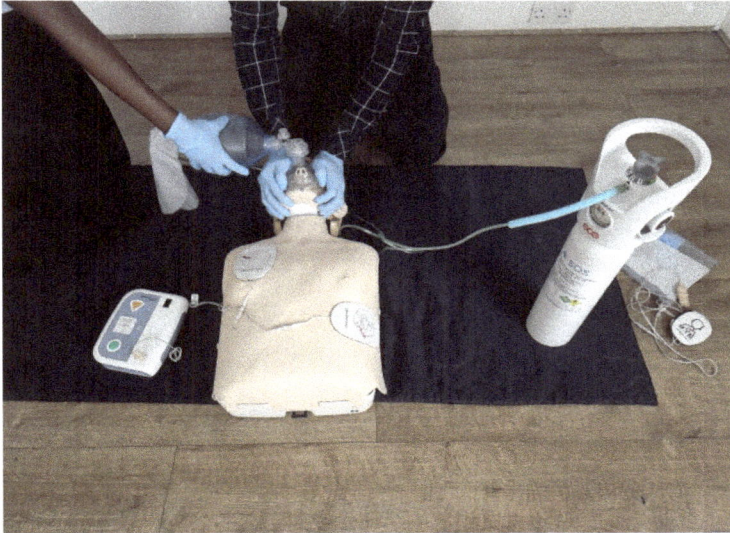

STEP 12

Bystander compressions: continuous chest compressions

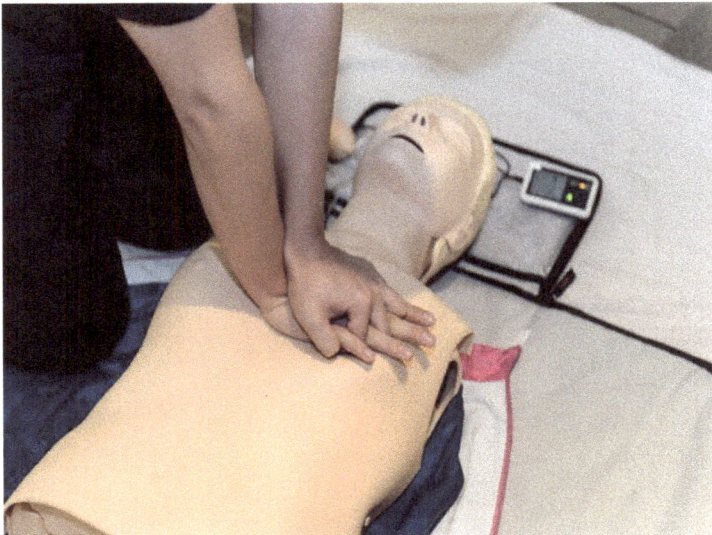

PERFORMING CPR ON A HEAVILY

PREGNANT WOMAN

So, when performing CPR on a heavily pregnant woman raise the right hip slightly so that the pregnant woman is leaning slightly to the left side. This has the effect of moving the uterus away from the blood vessel and creating an uninterrupted blood supply to the heart.

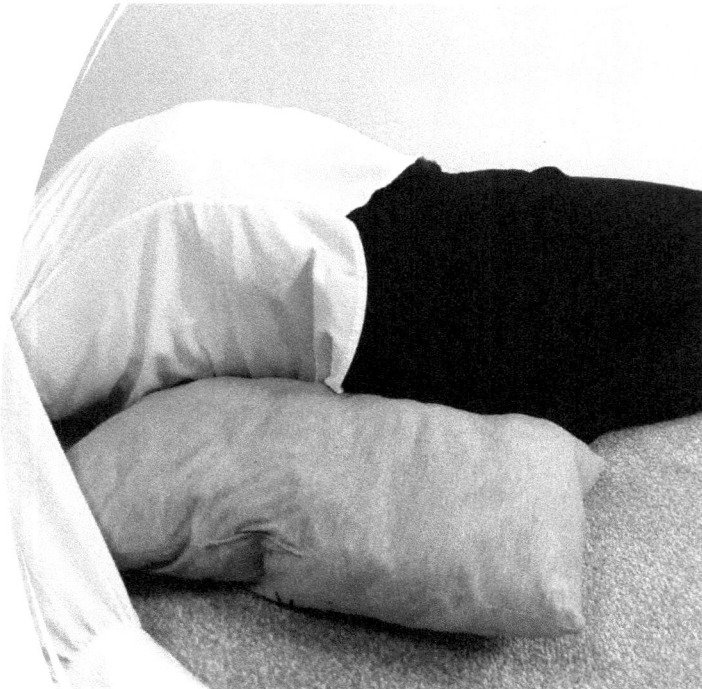

Child CPR

- Check for a response.
- Check the airway.
- Check if the patient is breathing and if not breathing call for help and commence CPR. Start with 5 rescue breaths, and 30 chest compressions. The next rescue breaths will be 2 rescue breaths followed by 30 chest compressions.
- Use a defibrillator if it is available. The use of a defibrillator must be a matter of priority.

Step 1

Make sure you check that you are safe and that the patient is not exposed to any danger.

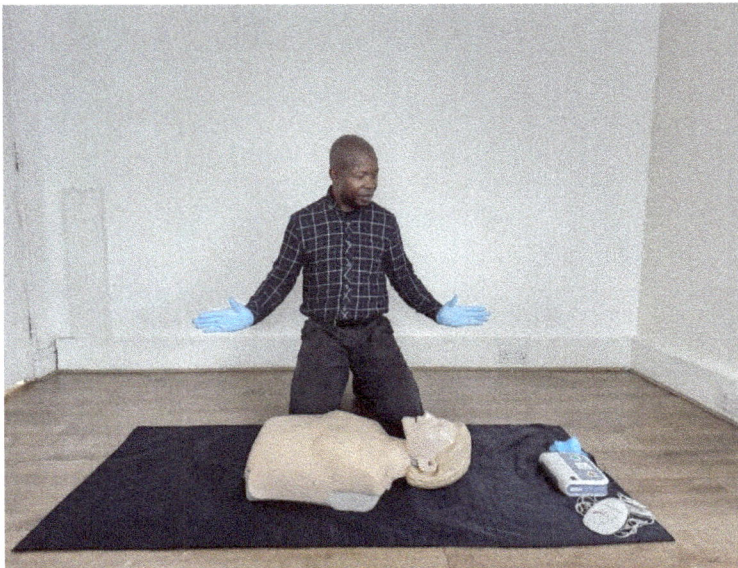

Step 2

Make sure you check if the patient is responsive. Two common ways of checking if a patient is responsive are to use both hands to tap on the patient's shoulder or squeeze on the patient's earlobes. Give a clear command like, " Wake up!" or "Open your eyes!"

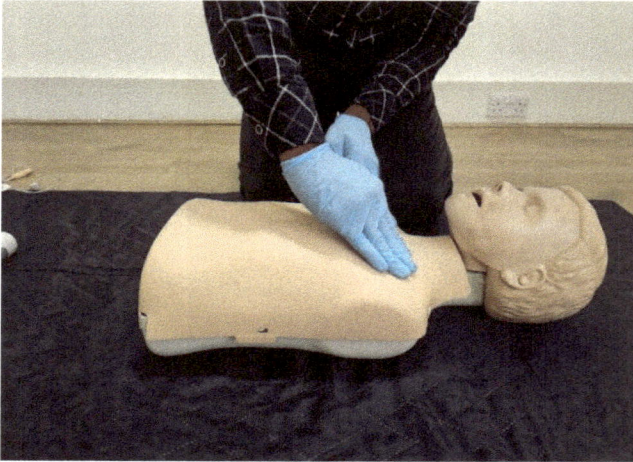

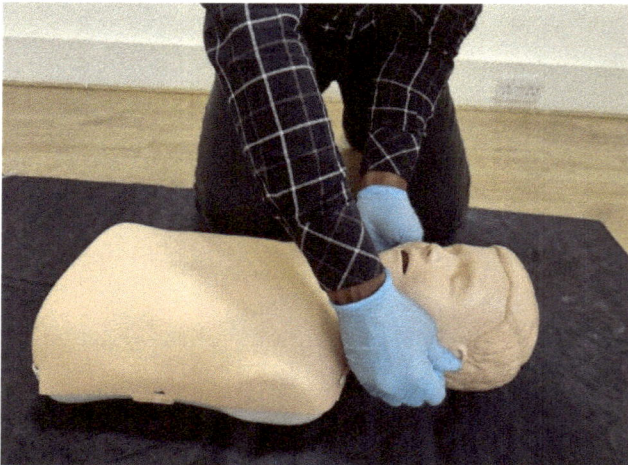

Step 3

Check if the airway is open by doing the head tilt and chin lift. Open the patient's mouth and check for any obstructions.

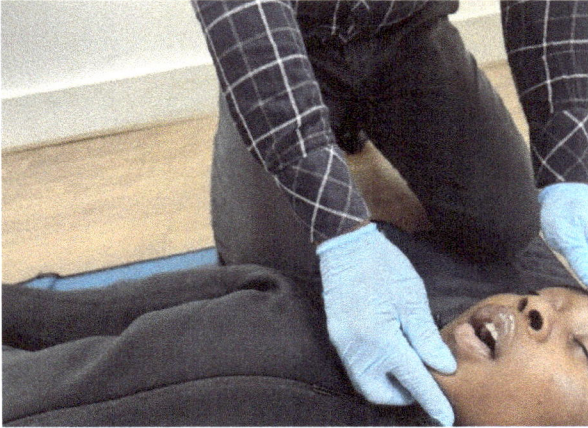

Step 4

Check whether the patient is breathing or not breathing. You should check for about 10 seconds.

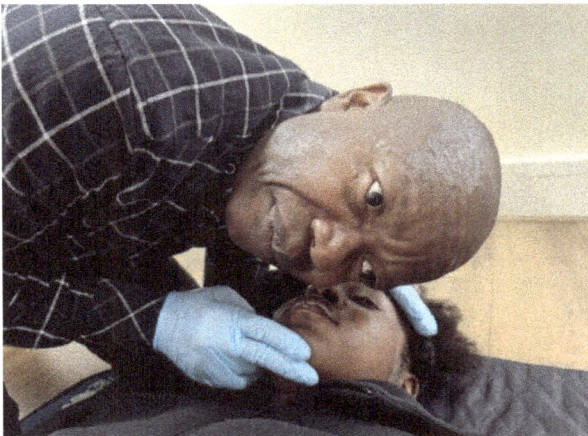

Step 5

Give 5 rescue breaths by sealing your mouth over the mouth of the child whilst squeezing the child 5 rescue breaths, and 30 chest compressions. The next rescue is mouth-to-mouth, mouth-to-face mask, mouth-to-pocket mask, or mouth-to-bag valve mask.

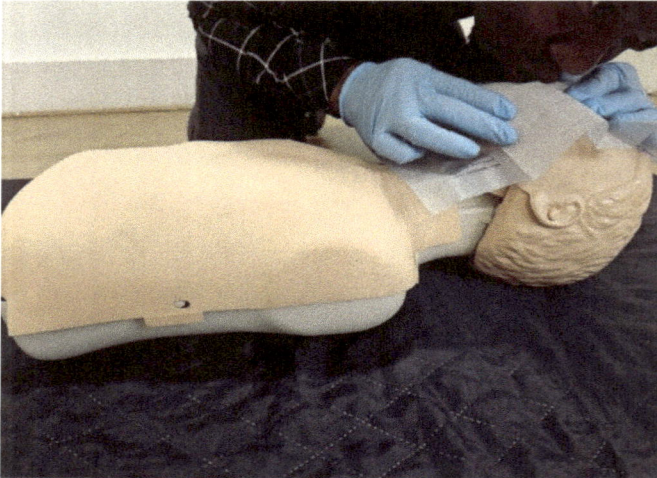

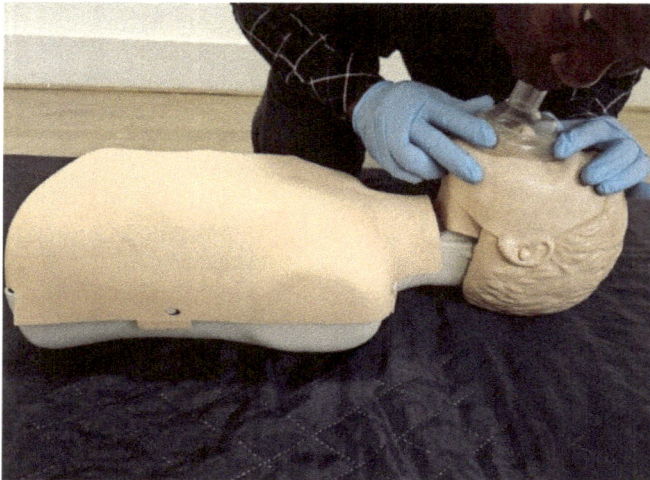

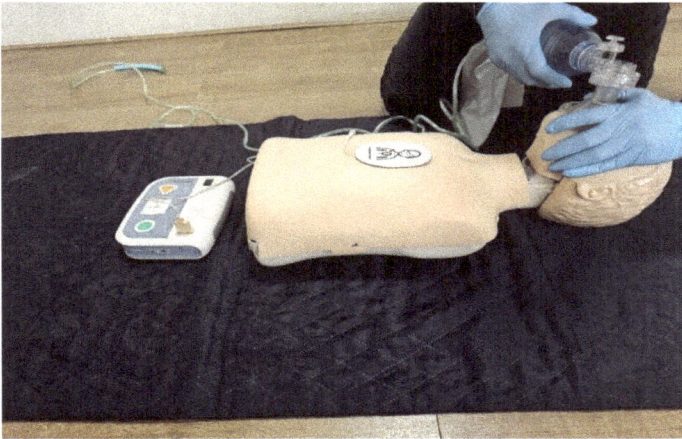

Step 6

Start chest compressions. As healthcare professionals, you are required to provide 15 chest compressions with one hand in the centre of the chest.

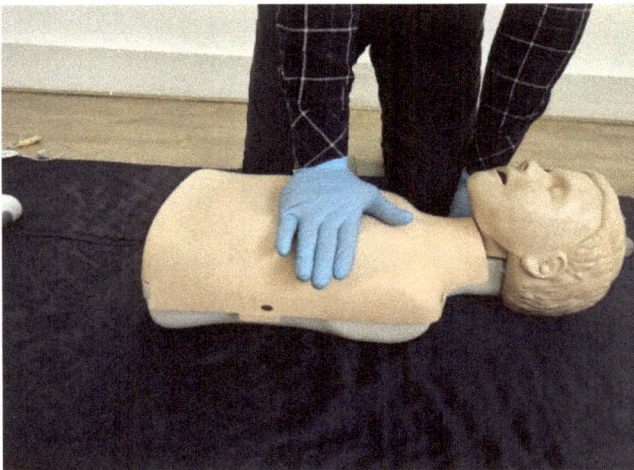

UNCONSCIOUS AND BREATHING

CHILD

STEP 1

check for danger.

STEP 2

Make sure you and the patient are safe.

PLACE ONE HAND ON THE FOREHEAD AND WITH TWO FINGERS TILT THE HEAD BACK SLIGHTLY

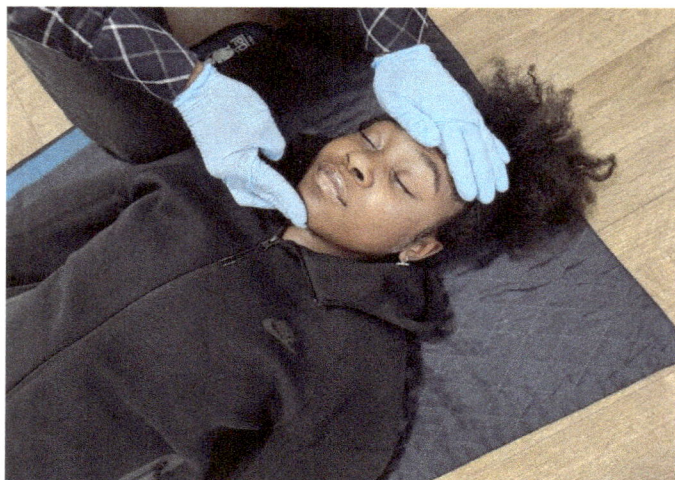

STEP 3

LEAN TOWARDS THE HEAD WITH YOUR CHEEK FACING THE CASUALTY in the centre of the chest.

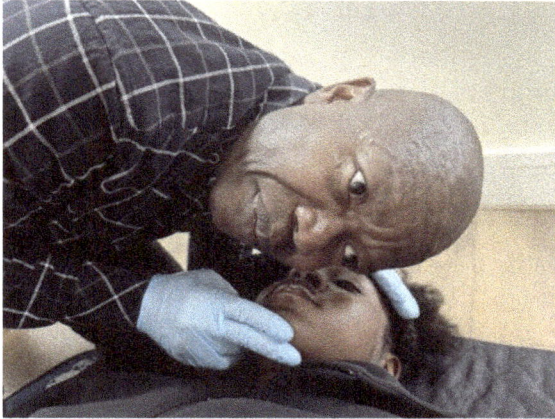

STEP 4

REACH FOR THE CASUALTY WITH YOUR CHEEK FACING THE CASUALTY IN RIGHT-ANGLED POSITION OR STRAIGHT.

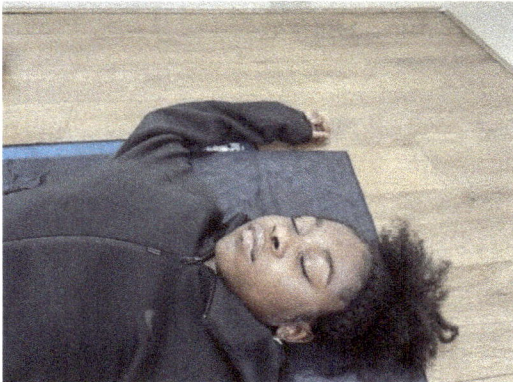

STEP 5

REACH OUT FOR THE CASUALTY YOUR CHEEK FAC FROM YOU AND PLACE IT ON HIS/HER CHEEK AND HOLD IT THERE.

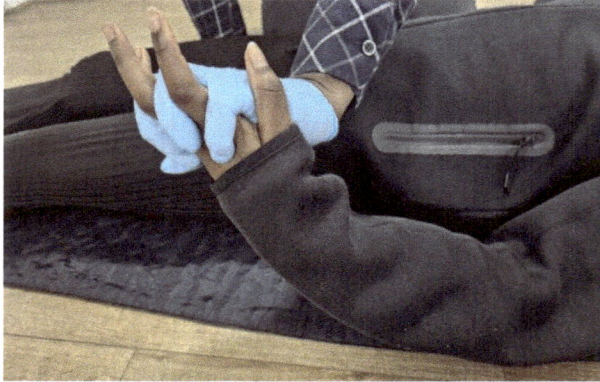

STEP 6

Place the back of the patient's hand on the cheek closest to you.

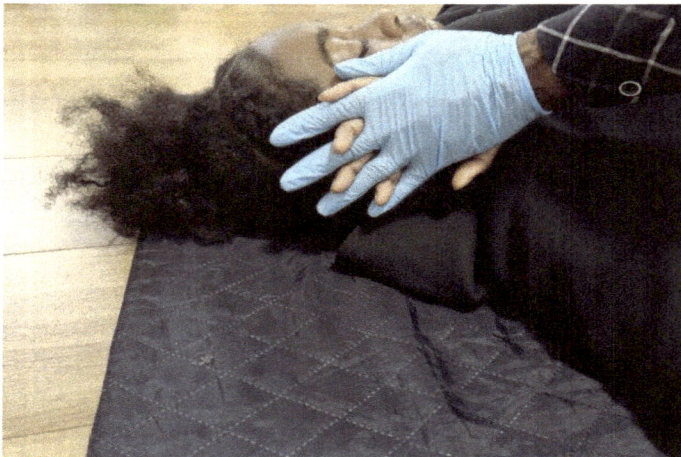

STEP 7

REACH FOR THE LEG FURTHEST FROM YOU AND RAISE IT FROM THE OUTER PART OF THE KNEE

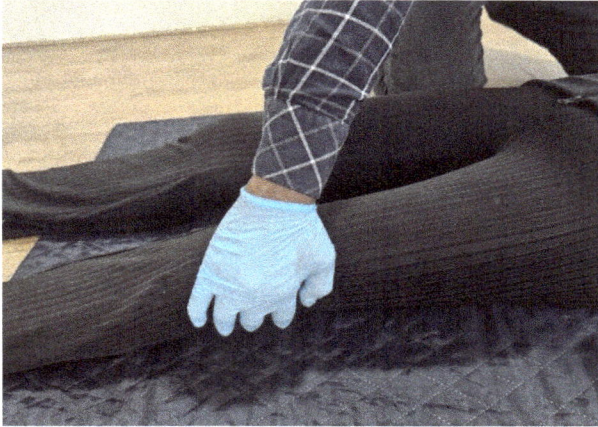

STEP 8

AREA MAKING SURE THE FEET ARE FIRMLY ON THE GROUND. AND LEAN THE CASUALTY TOWARDS YOU

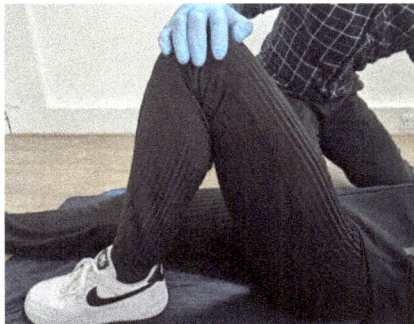

STEP 9

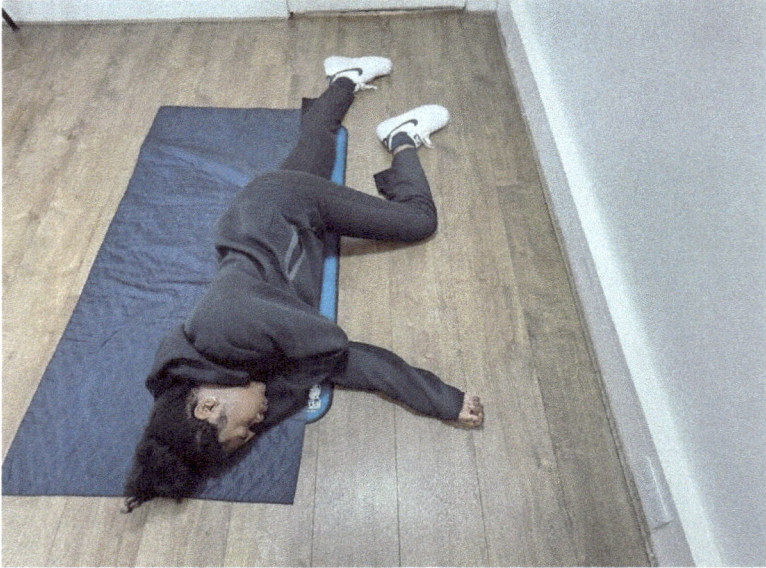

STEP 10

AGAIN, TILT THE CHIN UP TO CLEAR THE CASUALTY

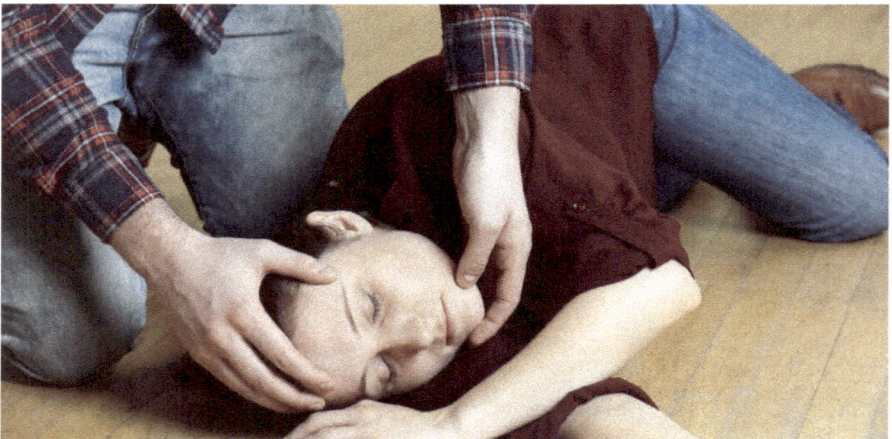

Infant CPR

Step 1

Check that you and the baby are safe and then check if the baby is responsive.

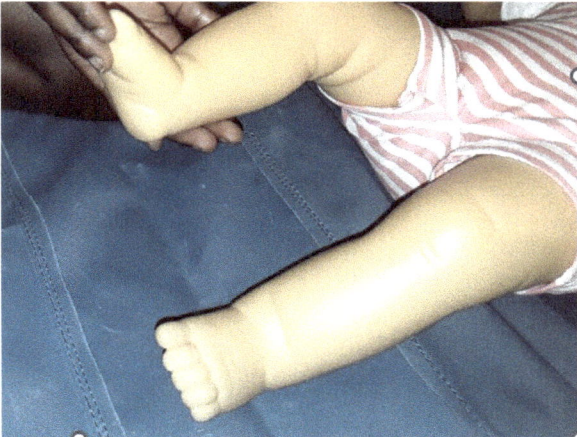

Step 2

Check airway- head tilt, chin lift.

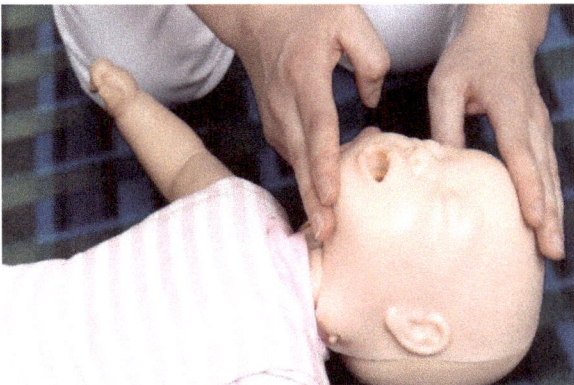

Step 3

Check breathing- look, listen, and feel.

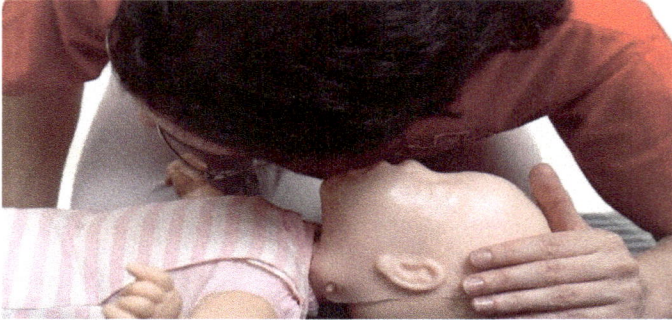

Step 4

Mouth-to-mouth rescue breath.

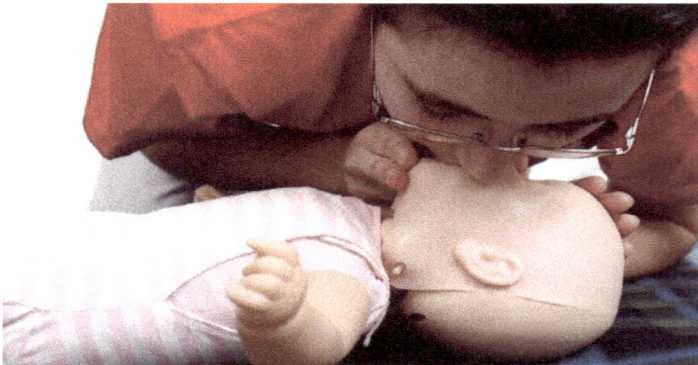

Step 5

Mouth-to-bag valve mask-one-person technique.

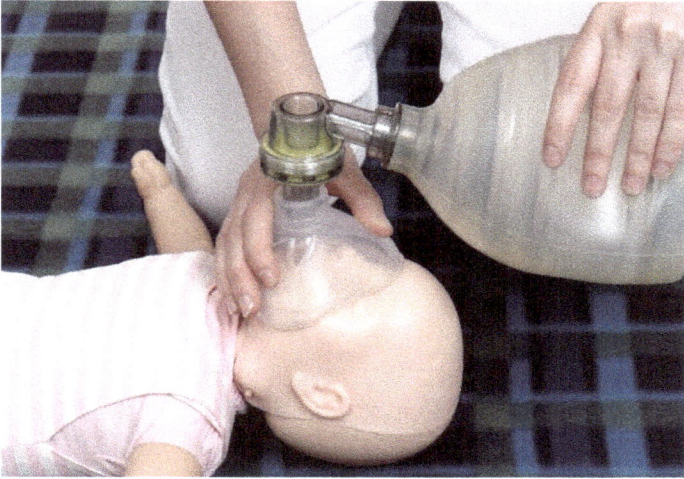

Step 6

Infant chest compressions on the CASUALTY

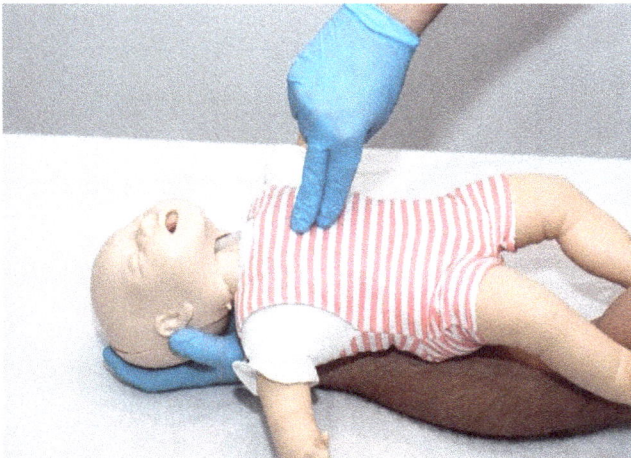

Infant compressions with two thumbs

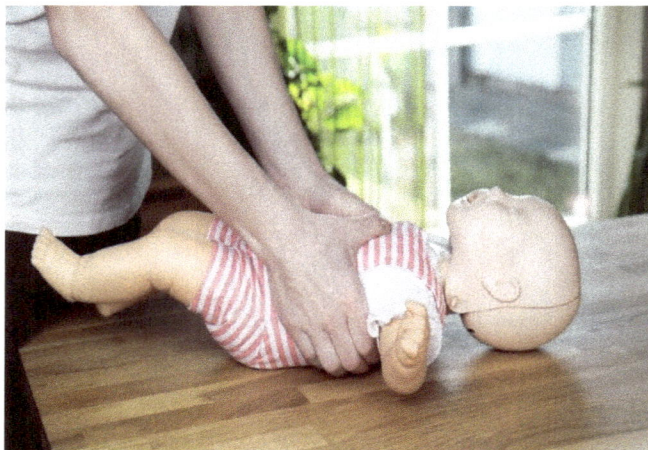

ADULT RECOVERY POSITION

STEP 1

- A safe and comfortable position aimed at opening the airway.

- Place the patient in a lateral position when unresponsive and breathing.

- Kneel beside the patient and straighten both legs.

- Place the arm nearest to you at a right angle to his body with his palm open.

- Bring the arm furthest from you and place the back of that hand on the patient's cheek nearest to you and hold it there.

- Whilst holding the patient hold it there. the back of that hand on the patient's chest, your hand on their knee and roll them over towards you. Ensure the head is tilted and adjust the hip and leg to bend at right angles.

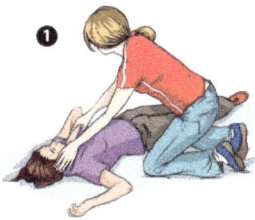

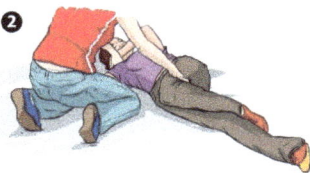

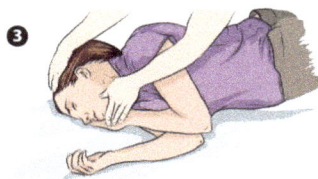

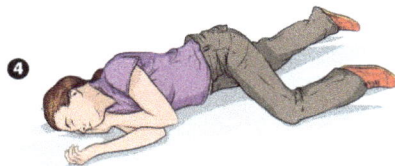

BABY RECOVERY POSITION

Step 1

Infant-Response check

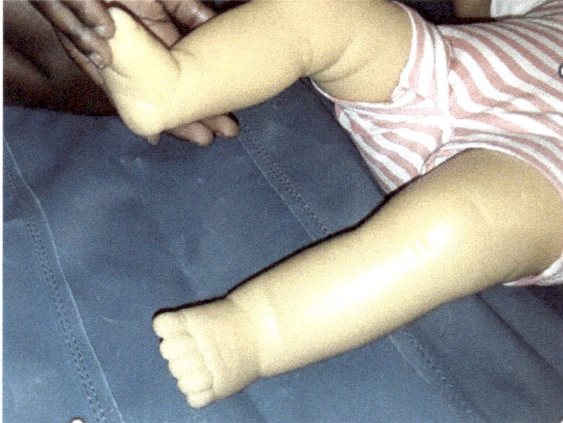

Step 2

Recovery Position-Infant- head tilt chin lift. Do not overextend the neck.

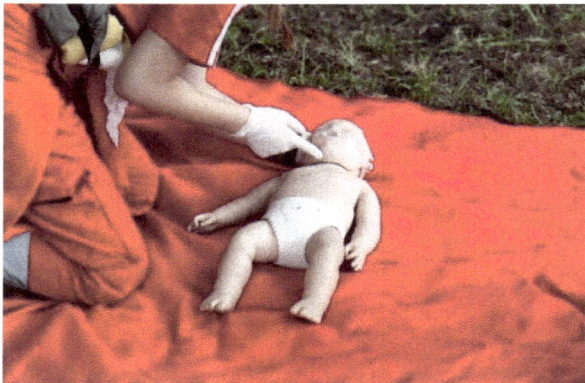

Step 3

Recovery Position-check baby and roll them

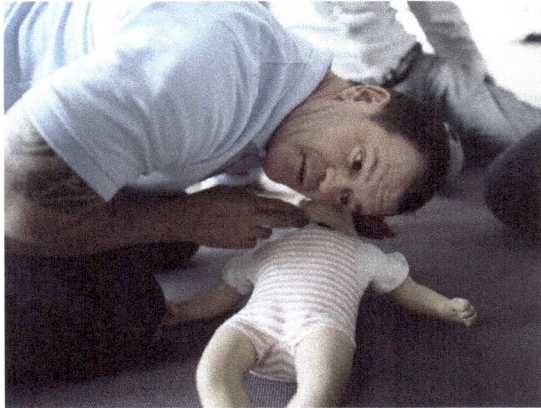

Step 4

Recovery position- Infant

Pick the baby up and hold him against your body with the head lower than the bottom to drain any fluid in the mouth and maintain a clear airway.

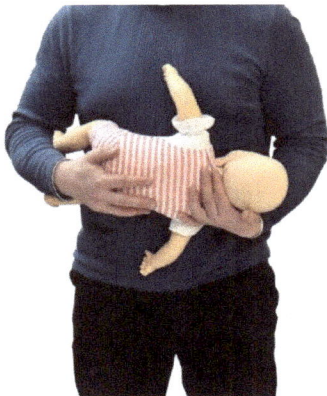

Asthma

EMERGENCY MEDICATIONS –SALBUTAMOL; TREATMENT FOR ASTHMA

ACTIONS

The management of asthma can take the form of inhaled bronchodilators and when those prove ineffective try intravenous (IV) medications. The aim of both medications is to reduce bronchospasm and inflammation of the lungs.

Salbutamol is a beta$_2$ adrenoreceptor stimulant drug. It is a bronchodilator which means that when administered through the mouth it opens the bronchial tubes (air passage) in the lungs.

The medication creates a relaxing effect on the muscles in the medium and smaller airways which are in spasm because of the patient's contact with a trigger. If used in combination with a nebuliser powered by oxygen they together smoothen and moisten the airway thereby creating a relaxing and relieving effect on the muscle. It acts within 5-6 minutes with a peak at around 15-20 minutes. The effects can last for about 4-6 hours.

PRESENTATION

Salbutamol nebuliser solution 5mg/2.5 ml

INDICATIONS

Salbutamol is used for acute asthma attacks in cases where normal inhaler therapy has not been effective in relieving the symptoms.

It is also used in cases of expiratory wheezing due to allergy, anaphylaxis, smoke inhalation, or other lower airway causes or worsening chronic obstructive pulmonary disease.

Respiratory distress.

CONTRA-INDICATIONS

None in emergency situations. Those with angioedema or patients with sensitivity to salbutamol. Use with caution when administering the medication to a patient who is a breastfeeding mother or patients with cardiovascular disorders or cardiac arrhythmias.

CAUTIONS

Salbutamol should be used with care in the following patients:

Hypertensive patients, angina, patients with overactive thyroid, a pregnant women in the late stages of pregnancy because the medication can lead to the relaxation of the uterus.

Taking salbutamol can also lead to severe hypertension in patients on beta blockers- drugs that prevent the stimulation of adrenergic receptors responsible for increased cardiac action, used to control heart rhythm, angina attack, and high blood pressure.

In cases of patients with COPD, reduce nebulisation to no more than 6 minutes.

SIDE EFFECTS

Tremor, (shaking), Tachycardia (fast heartbeat), palpitations, headache, feeling of tension, muscle cramps, rash, and peripheral vasodilation.

DOSAGE AND ADMINISTRATION

Adult-5 mg/2.5ml nebulised 5-6 minutes. Give medication every 5 minutes intervals until the patient recovers or the emergency services arrive.

SALBUTAMOL AEROSOL INHALER (100 MICROGRAMS/ metered inhalation)

Medication	Age of patient	Route of administration	Dosage	Duration
Salbutamol Aerosol inhaler	Child under the age of 3 years	By aerosol inhalation through a spacer	2-10 puffs	Repeated 10 to 20 minutes or if necessary
Salbutamol Aerosol inhaler	Adults	By aerosol inhalation through a spacer	2-10 puffs	Repeated 10 to 20 minutes or if necessary

SALBUTAMOL NEBULISER SOLUTION (1mg/mL, 2mg/mL)

Medication	Age of patient	Route of administration	Dosage	Duration
Salbutamol Nebuliser solution	Child under 4 years	Inhalation of oxygen driven nebuliser	2.5mg	Repeated every 20 - 30 minutes or as required
Salbutamol Nebuliser solution	Child 5-11 years	Inhalation through a nebuliser	2.5-5mg	Repeated 10 to 20-30minutes or if necessary
Salbutamol Nebuliser solution	Child 12-17 years	Inhalation through a nebuliser	5mg	Repeated 10 to 20-30minutes or if necessary
Salbutamol Nebuliser solution	Adult	Inhalation through a nebuliser	5mg	Repeated 10 to 20-30minutes or if necessary

TERBULINE SULFATE 2.5mg/mL (This can be given instead of Salbutamol)

Medication	Age of patient	Route of administration	Dosage	Duration
Terbutaline nebuliser solution	Under 4 years old	By inhalation of nebulised solution preferably through oxygen driven nebuliser if available	5mg	Repeated every 20-30 minutes or as necessary
Terbutaline nebuliser solution	5-11 years	By inhalation of nebulised solution preferably through oxygen driven nebuliser if available	5-10mg	Repeated every 20-30 minutes or as necessary
Terbutaline nebuliser solution	12-17 years	By inhalation of nebulised solution preferably through oxygen driven nebuliser	10mg	Repeated every 20-30 minutes or as necessary

		if available		
Terbut aline nebulis er solutio n	Adult	By inhalation of nebulised solution preferably through oxygen driven nebuliser if available	10mg	Repeated every 20-30 minutes or as necessary

In addition to either Salbutamol, Terbutaline, Prednisolone tablets, prednisolone soluble tablets, or hydrocortisone (sodium succinate)

PREDNISOLONE

Prednisolone tablets or prednisolone soluble tablets

Medicat ion	Age of patient	Route of administration	Dosag e	Duration
Predniso lone	Child under 11 years old	Mouth	1- 2mg /kg (max 40 mg)	Once daily for up to 3 days or longer if necessary If the child has been administered oral

				corticosteroid for a few days then give prednisolone 2mg/kg (maximum 60 mg/kg) once daily
Predniso lone	Child 12-17 years	mouth	40-50mg	Once daily for at least 5 days
Predniso lone	Adult	mouth	40-50mg	Once daily for at least 5 days

HYDROCORTISONE (sodium succinate)

Medication	Age of patient	Route of administration	Dosage	Duration
Hydrocortisone	Child under 17years old	Intravenous injection	4mg /kg (max 100 mg)	Every 6 hours until a change to oral prednisolone is possible
Hydrocortisone	Child 1 year or below	Intravenous injection	25mg	
Hydrocortisone	Child 2 - 4years	Intravenous injection	50mg	
Hydrocortisone	5-17 years	Intravenous injection	100mg	
Hydrocortisone	Adult	Intravenous injection	100mg	Every 6 hours until change to oral prednisolone is possible

IPRATROPIUM BROMIDE (Atrovent)

Medication	Age of patient	Route of administration	Dosage	Duration
Ipratropium Bromide	Child under 11years old	Inhalation through a nebuliser (Preferably through an oxygen-driven nebuliser)	250 Micrograms	Repeated every 20-30 minutes for the first 2 hours. Thereafter to be repeated 4-6 hours as if needed
Ipratropium Bromide	Child 12-17 years-	Inhalation through a nebuliser (Preferably through an oxygen-driven nebuliser)	500 micrograms	Repeated every 4-6 hours if necessary
Ipratropium	Adult	Inhalation	500microg	Every- 6

Bromide		through a nebuliser (Preferably through an oxygen-driven nebuliser)	rams	hours

Guidelines for the Management of asthma in a dental practice[4]

Administer salbutamol with a spacer device one puff at a time.

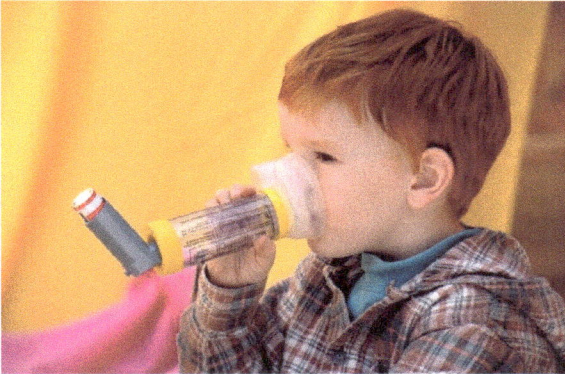

Spacer device

Give another puff every 60 seconds up to a maximum of 10 puffs.

Follow the patient's own personalised action plan. They should be advised to always have it with them.

---

[4] British Thoracic Society. BTS/SIGN British Guideline on the Management of Asthma. 2019. Available online at https://www.brit-thoracic.org.uk/quality-improvement/guidelines/asthma/ (accessed April 2020).

SEIZURES

This is an abnormal electrical discharge in the brain.

These are caused by abnormal electrical activity in the brain. There are many types of seizures, but each type depends on the part of the brain that is affected. However, bilateral tonic-clonic seizures are the most common type of seizures. It starts with the tonic phase (which is when the body stiffens and then gives way to the clonic stage which is when the body shakes vigorously. Typically, the eyes open, and the patient is unresponsive to commands, nor do they respond to any sensory stimuli (JRCALC). BTCS will normally stop after 90 seconds after they start. Often characterised by patients becoming confused/ and or drowsy

Epilepsy is a chronic disorder in which patients are at risk of unprovoked seizures and they are usually caused by.

o   Stroke

•   Alcohol

•   Hypoglycaemia

•   Drug overdose.

•   infection

OTHER SIGNS

- Patient eyes open and the white part of the eyes roll to the top of the head.
- They are unresponsive to commands or sensory stimuli.
- Will generally stop about 90 seconds after it began.
- Confusion afterwards.
- Drowsy (JRCALC)

Q1   Convulsive Status Epilepticus

This is a tonic-clonic seizure that has not stopped after five minutes or a series of such seizures without any recovery in-between which lasts for 5 minutes or more. This is a medical emergency.

FOCAL SEIZURE (Aura)-This is a seizure that starts in one part of the brain and spreads to the other part of the brain to cause a tonic-clonic seizure. Focal seizures should be treated as tonic-clonic seizures if they last for more than 10 minutes and there is an impaired level of consciousness. There is a risk of long-term damage if the focal seizures continue for more than 60 minutes (JRCALC)

PHASES OF SEIZURES

BEGINNING PHASE –

PRODROME STAGE—

Some people can tell that the seizure is about to start. This may be signs felt hours or days before but not everyone will experience this phase.

COMMON SIGNS

- Mood changes
- Anxiety
- Feeling light-headed
- Difficulty sleeping
- Difficulty staying awake
- Behavioural changes

AURA

It is that sense that you get that something is about to happen.

This is the early part of the seizure.

Symptoms

- Feeling of déjà vu (a sense that something has happened before when in fact it has not)
- Jamais vu (a feeling that you are seeing something that you know

well for the first time)

- Odd smells, sounds, or tastes.

- Dizziness

- Vision difficulties

- Numbness or 'pins and needles in parts of the body

- Nausea

- Headache

- Panic

- Feelings of intense fear (Heart Foundation)

MIDDLE (ICTAL) PHASE

This is the time from the beginning of the seizure to the end of the seizure. This is when there is intense electrical activity in the brain. Common signs

- Loss of awareness
- Memory lapse
- Difficulty hearing, twitching, feeling confused, odd smells or sounds or tastes, saying strange words, loss of muscle control, repeated lip smacking or chewing,

END PHASE (POST ICTAL PHASE)

This usually occurs after the active(ictal) part of the seizure. This is also called the recovery stage.

Common signs

- Confusion
- Lack of consciousness
- Tiredness
- Exhaustion
- Headache
- Loss of bladder or bowel control
- Fear and anxiety.
- Frustration
- Shame and embarrassment
- Thirst
- Nausea

Weakness in parts of the body (Epilepsy foundation)

ASSESSMENT AND MANAGEMENT OF EPILEPTIC SEIZURES

Position—Ensure the casualty and you are safe. Place the casualty in the recovery position to maintain a clear airway and prevent him from choking on his vomit.

History—Take the history of the illness. Are there any witnesses? Estimate the length of the seizures. Has the patient been diagnosed with epilepsy, or is it an isolated case/cluster of seizures? Were there any symptoms preceding the seizures? Was there any pregnancy?

History of diabetes/hypertension/heart disease/medication use/alcohol intake.

Airway—Consider using the oropharyngeal airway, but not if they do not tolerate it. Alternatively, use a nasal pharyngeal airway, but do not use it if there is a basal skull fracture or facial trauma.

Breathing-assess the breathing rate and quality of the patient's breathing.

If the patient has a tonic-clonic seizure, administer oxygen at a rate of fifteen litres per minute. Aim for oxygen saturation of 94-98 % or 88-92% if the patient has COPD.

If pulse oximetry is low or ETCO2 is high then use a bag valve mask (BVM) to conduct ventilation where possible with the aid of an airway adjunct

Do not delay the administration of medication during the convulsion as the administration of medication has been proven to improve ventilation.

Injuries– look out for them eg head injury/incontinence-urinary incontinence occurs in patients with epileptic seizures/ look out for a non-blanching rash which indicates meningitis.

Examine the abdomen of female patients for pregnancy and eclampsia.

Description of the seizure– write down the characteristics of the convulsion.

TREATEMENT

BUCCAL MIDAZOLAM OR DIAZEPAM

Treatment with diazepam

This medication should only be used for patients with ongoing convulsions. A patient should be given diazepam if they have seizures lasting more than 5 minutes or more. Or if they have three or more convulsions in an hour or those who are currently convulsing

PSYCHOGENIC NONEPILEPTIC SEIZURES

These are attacks that may look like epileptic seizures but are not caused by abnormal brain electrical discharges. They are usually the result of psychological distress.

CAUSES OF PNES

traumatic events

Divorce

Death of a loved one

Sudden change

The best way to diagnose PNES is through video EEG (electroencephalograph) monitoring. This records what you are doing or experiencing on videotape while an EEG test records your brainwaves.[5]

SIGNS AND SYMPTOMS

- Fluctuating intensity/location
- Brief pauses, tremors, or slow flexion/extension movement
- Arms and legs are often not synchronised.
- Convulsions may move from one body area to another.
- May respond in one way to speech or NPA insertion.
- Tongue biting
- Eyes are mostly shut.
- Mouth often shut.
- Pupils reacting
- May conduct purposeful movements.
- Normal spo2, no cyanosis, hyperventilation
- May be prolonged, or may be 3 minutes.
- Pelvic thrusting is common.
- Arching of the head, neck, and spine is common.

---

[5] **Selim R Benbadis, MD** Professor, Director of Comprehensive Epilepsy Program, Departments of Neurology and Neurosurgery, Tampa General Hospital, University of South Florida Morsani College of Medicine

- Side-to-side movement of the head

- Crying during or after a convulsion

- Big toe flexed down (JRCALC)

PNES –POST ICTAL

The post-ictal stage usually happens after the active (ictal) part of the seizure. This is also referred to as the recovery stage.

COMMON SIGNS OF THE PNES POST- ICTAL PHASE

- Rapid end to convulsion
- Rapid post-ictal recovery
- Normal post-ictal breathing

PNES: HISTORY

Onset over 15 years

Recurrent 'status epilepticus' (a misdiagnosis)

PTSD

Buccal Midazolam –emergency medication for patients with prolonged convulsions

Presentation

Pre-filled syringes of 2.5mg, 5mg, 7.5mg or 10mg

Indications

The medications can be given to patients with convulsions lasting 5 minutes or more or who have had 3 or 4 convulsions within an hour and are still convulsing.

Also, to be administered where convulsions have persisted 10 minutes after the initial dose of the medication.

This medication requires a PGD (Patients Group Directions) before it can be administered unless the patient has his own prescribed supply. PGDs are a set of written instructions to help supply or administer medicines to patients in planned circumstances. (Medicines and Healthcare Products Regulatory Agencies –"Patients Group directions-who can use them": updated 4th December 2017)

Examples of those who can administer or supply drugs under PGDs are Dental Hygienists, Dental Therapists, Pharmacists, Midwives, Nurses, Paramedics, and Physiotherapists. Please see the directions for the full lists of healthcare professionals not mentioned here permitted to use PGDs.

Cautions

The medication can lead to respiratory arrest due to respiratory depression. Patients likely to be affected by this are children, chronically ill patients, and patients 60 years old and over. Particularly vulnerable are patients who are drunk or who have ingested other sedative drugs.

Contraindications

None

Side effects

Confusion, amnesia, hypotension, deteriorating levels of consciousness, and respiratory depression.

Seizures lasting more than 5 minutes.

Diazepam Rectal solution (2mg/mL, 4mg/mL)

Medication	Age of patient	Route of administration	Dosage	Duration	Body weight
Diazepam Rectal solution	Neonates	Rectum	1.25-2.5mg	Repeated once after 5-10 minutes if necessary	
Diazepam Rectal Solution	1 month-1 year	Rectum	5mg	Repeated once after 5-10 minutes if necessary	

Diazepam Rectal solution	2-11 years	Rectum	5-10mg	Repeated once after 5-10 minutes
Diazepam Rectal solution	12-17 years	Rectum	10-20g	Repeated once after 5-10 minutes

Diazepam Rectal solution	Adult	Rectum	10-20g	Repeated once after 5-10 minutes
Diazepam Rectal solution	Elderly	Rectum	10mg	Repeated once after 5-10 minutes

MIDAZOLAM OR MUCOSAL SOLUTION

Medication	Age of patient	Route of administration	Dosage	Duration	Body weight
Midazolam Oro mucosal solution	Neonates	Buccal administration	300 microgram/kg	Repeated once after 5-10 minu	

				tes if nece ssary	
Midazola m Oro mucosal solution	Child-1-2 months	Buccal administration	300 microg rams/k g (Maxi mum 2.5 mg)	Repe ated once after 5-10 minu tes if nece ssary	
Midazola m Oro mucosal solution	Child 3 months- 11 months	Buccal administration	2.5mg	Repe ated once after 5-10 minu tes	
Midazola m Oro mucosal solution	1-4years	Buccal administration	5mg	Repe ated once after 5-10	

				minutes	
Midazolam Oro mucosal solution	5-9 years	Buccal administration	7.5mg	Repeated once after 5-10 minutes	
Midazolam Oro mucosal solution	10-17 years	Buccal Administration	10mg	Repeated once after 5-10 minutes	
Midazolam Oro mucosal solution	Adult	Buccal administration	10 mg	Repeated once after 5-10 minutes	

Positional Treatment

Recovery Position

When the patient's seizure stops, he should be placed in the recovery position.

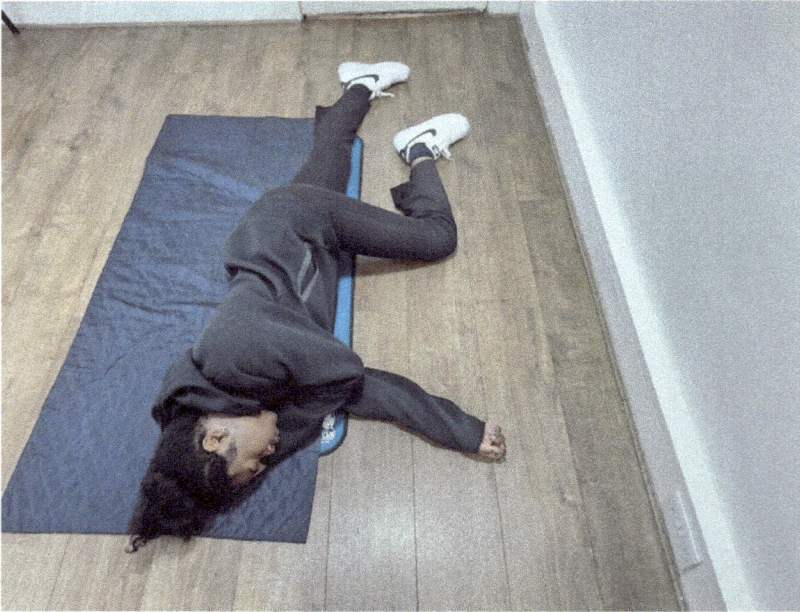

NICE GUIDELINES TO MANAGING

EPILETIC SEIZURES.

1. All patients with epilepsy should have a **personalised care plan** which should be brought with them to the dental appointment and must be followed if the patient has an epileptic seizure at the practice.

2. Buccolam contains Midazolam hydrochloride 5mg/1mL in pre-filled oral syringes of 2.5 mg, 5mg, 7.5 mg, and 10mg.

3. Epistatus contains midazolam maleate 10mg/1mL. It is prepared in 5mL bottle with 4 oral syringes in the package. It is available in pre-filled oral syringes of 2.5 mg, 5mg, 7.5 mg, and 10 mg.

STROKE

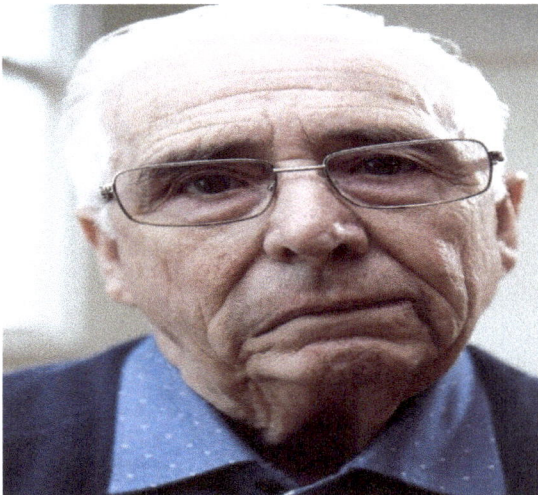

Transient Ischaemic Attack (TIA)

Stroke can be caused by either a blood clot in one or more blood vessels supplying blood to the brain or a rupture in the blood vessels in the brain.

Stroke is not age-specific. It can happen to anyone of any age. Time is of the essence. The speed of recovery depends on how soon the patient arrives in the hospital and receives urgent treatment.

Signs and symptoms

1. Numbness or weakness of the face, arms, or legs on either left or right side of the body
2. Sudden onset of
3. Seizures, syncope, sepsis, hypoglycemia
4. confusion, difficulty speaking, difficulty swallowing, and inability or difficulty understanding speech.
5. Sudden blurred vision in one or both eyes
6. Lack of coordination, loss of gait, and difficulty walking
7. Severe headache
8. Dizziness, nausea, or vomiting
9. Sudden neck pain or neck stiffness

TIA (Transient Ischaemic Attack)

This is a temporary disruption of blood to part of the brain[6]

Signs and symptoms

Face- Droopy face, difficulty in smiling

Arm – cannot lift one or both arms.

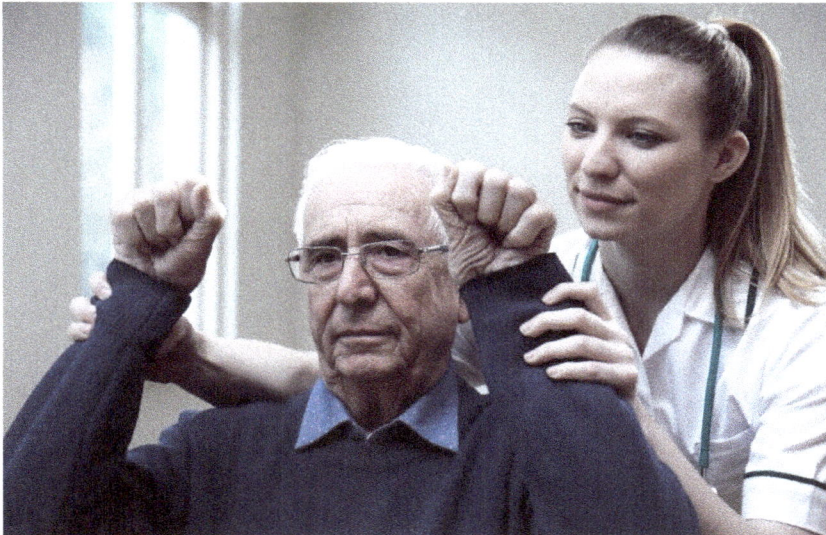

Speech – slurred speech

[6] **Transient ischaemic attack (TIA) - NHS (www.nhs.uk)**

Treatment of Stroke and TIA

- Call 99/112
- Monitor airway and breathing.
- If unconscious, place in a recovery position
- If the patient is conscious, make sure he lies down with his head and shoulder raised.

ANAPHYLACTIC REACTIONS

Anaphylactic reactions within a dental practice may be triggered by the administration of drugs or contact with latex gloves, additives used in a dental practice, and excipients in medicines.

SIGNS

Respiratory arrests triggering cardiac arrest.

Flushing and pallor

Abdominal pain, vomiting, and diarrhoea.

Urticaria

Rhinitis

Conjunctivitis

Upper airway oedema and bronchospasm leading to stridor and wheezing.

ADRENALINE

TREATMENT FOR ANAPHYLAXIS

Adrenaline also known as epinephrine is a hormone produced by the adrenal glands during stressful or emotional situations. It works by stimulating part of the nervous system called the sympathetic nervous system which controls the unconscious actions of the body. In emergencies, it should be used to treat anaphylaxis and provide relief in acute asthma where there is bronchospasm.

Get the patient to lie in a supine position with both legs raised and administer oxygen at a rate of 10 litres/minute.

PRESENTATION

Pre-filled syringe or ampoules containing 1 milligram of adrenaline (epinephrine) in 1 ml (1:1000)

INDICATIONS

Anaphylaxis

Life-threatening asthma with failing ventilation and worsening despite nebuliser therapy.

CAUTION

Do not administer IV adrenaline in case of anaphylaxis.

DOSAGE AND ADMINISTRATION

FIRST DOSE

0-5 YEARS-150 MICROGRAMS

6-11 YEARS-300 MICROGRAMS

12-ADULT– 500 MICROGRAMS

SECOND DOSE

0-5 YEARS-150 MICROGRAMS

6-11 YEARS-300 MICROGRAMS

12-ADULT– 500 MICROGRAMS

Repeat every 5 minutes subsequently.

MAX DOSE: NO LIMIT

Use of the Adrenaline Auto-Injector

EMERADE

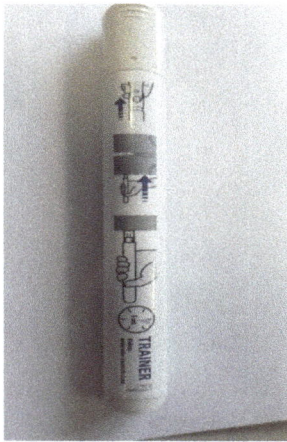

STEP 1

Remove the needle shield.

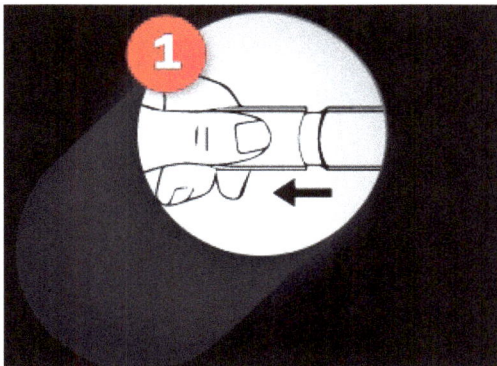

STEP 2

Press the pen against the outer thigh.

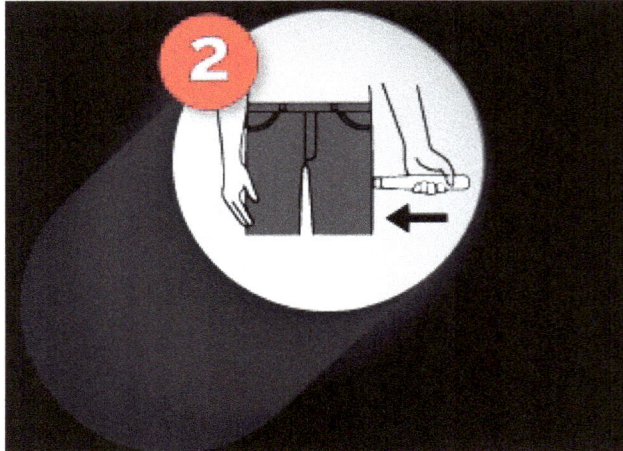

STEP 3

Hold for 5 seconds and message the injection site gently.

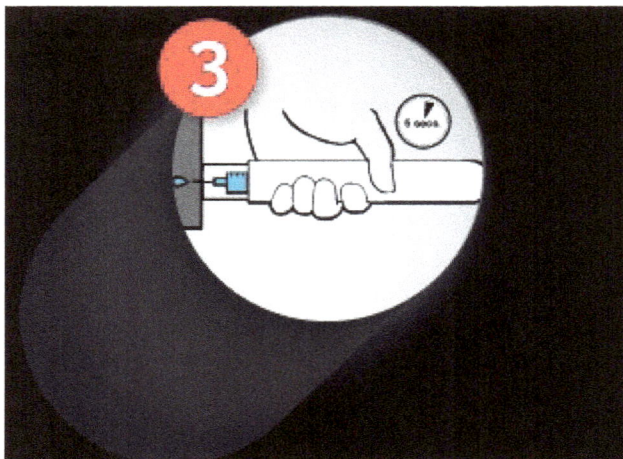

Call 999/112.

Even if the casualty begins to feel better and specifically.

5-15 minutes after the first dose

After 5-15 minutes, if the first does not work, administer a second one if available. If more than two is necessary, this must only be administered under medical supervision.

EPIPEN-

HOW TO USE THE EPIPEN

STEP 1

Form your fist around the EpiPen and remove the safety cap by pulling it straight up.

STEP 2

Swing and push the orange part of the auto-injector firmly against the anterolateral thigh until it "clicks." Hold the injection in place for 3 seconds. Count "1,2,3" slowly.

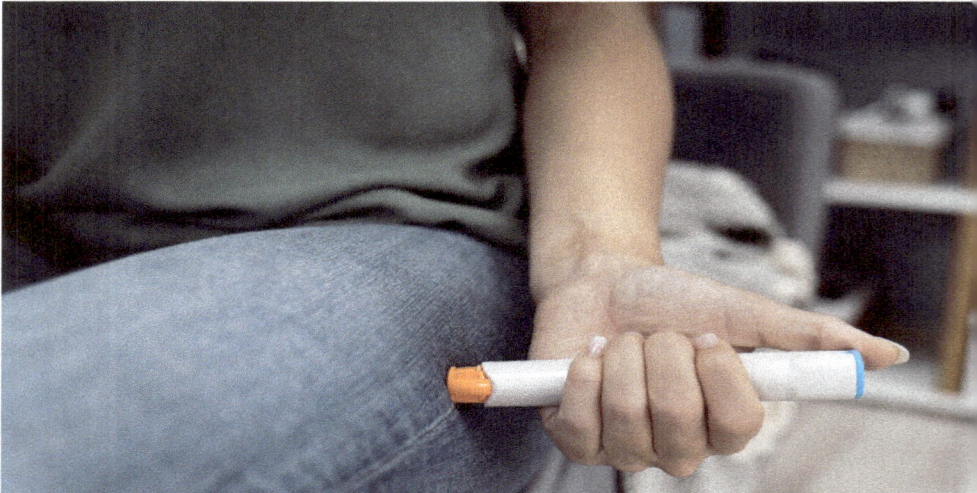

STEP 3

After injection, the orange cover automatically extends to ensure the needle is never exposed.

STEP 4

Isolate the casualty from the trigger.

Make sure the casualty is isolated from the trigger. For example, if a bee has stung the casualty, remove the stinger stuck to the skin.

RECOMMENDED NEEDLE LENGTH

The resuscitation council recommends that the length should be 25mm for all ages. This is based on a recommendation from Public Health England.[7]

Dental practice should have adrenaline 1:1000 (1mg/ml) ampoules in their emergency drugs kit. Anaphylaxis packs should have the following:

- Adrenaline 1:1000 ampoules x 2

- Blue 23G 25 mm needles x 4

- Graduated 1 ml syringes x 4.

Some dental practices prefer pre-filled syringes. The advantage of the pre-filled syringes is that they prevent the need to draw the medication from an ampoule.

The injection should be administered in the anterolateral aspect of the middle third of the thigh, but if that is not possible then administered on the arm.

---

[7] Public Health England. Immunisation against infectious disease. 2014. Available online at https://www.gov.uk/government/collections/immunisation-against-infectious-disease-the-green-book (accessed April 2020).

ADRENAL INSUFFICIENCY

This occurs because of insufficient production of steroid hormones in the adrenal cortex of the adrenal glands. A survey conducted in the UK in 2013 concluded that 8% of patients had developed adrenal crises whilst being treated in a dental practice.[8] This condition normally flows from prolonged use of oral corticosteroids and can persist for years after discontinuing the treatment.

" Life-threatening symptoms such as severe dehydration, hypotension, hypovolaemic shock, altered consciousness, seizures, stroke, or cardiac arrest may develop; if left untreated, adrenal crisis may lead to death or permanent disability."[9]

Signs

Ask the patient if they have a steroid emergency card.

Hypotension due to prolonged physiological stress.

MINOR DENTAL PROCEDURES (SCALE AND POLISH, REPLACEMENT FILLING)

---

[8] Addison's Self-Help Group. Adrenal Crisis Can Kill. 2020. Available at https://www.addisonsdisease.org.uk/emergency (accessed June 2020).

[9] https://bnf.nice.org.uk/treatment-summaries/adrenal-insufficiency/

The patient should be advised to take an extra dose of glucocorticoid.

One hour before the procedure.

The patient should be prescribed steroid supplementation before and 24 hours afterward.

COMPLEX DENTAL PROCEDURES (ROOT CANAL WORK UNDER LOCAL ANAESTHETICS)

This can be avoided by providing a patient with corticosteroids (Hydrocortisone) prophylactically before treatment. Physiological stress is in dental that requires increased steroid dose. Surgical extractions and implant placement should be considered a risk.

Advise all patients with adrenal insufficiency to bring their hydrocortisone injection kit and their personalised adrenal crisis letter to every appointment.

ADRENAL CRISIS DURING TREATMENT IN A DENTAL PRACTICE

CALL 999/112 and tell them your patient is having an "Addisonian crisis."

If the patient has an emergency hydrocortisone kit, administer intramuscular hydrocortisone.

RECOMMENDED DOSE

ADULT-100mg

CHILDREN-6 Years or older-50-100mg

INFANTS- Up to one year old- 25mg

The Addison clinical advisory panel advises increasing the patient's dose of steroids for patients with Addison's disease before they undergo any significant dental treatment under local anesthetic. Addison's disease is a condition that happens when the body does not produce enough of certain hormones.

OXYGEN

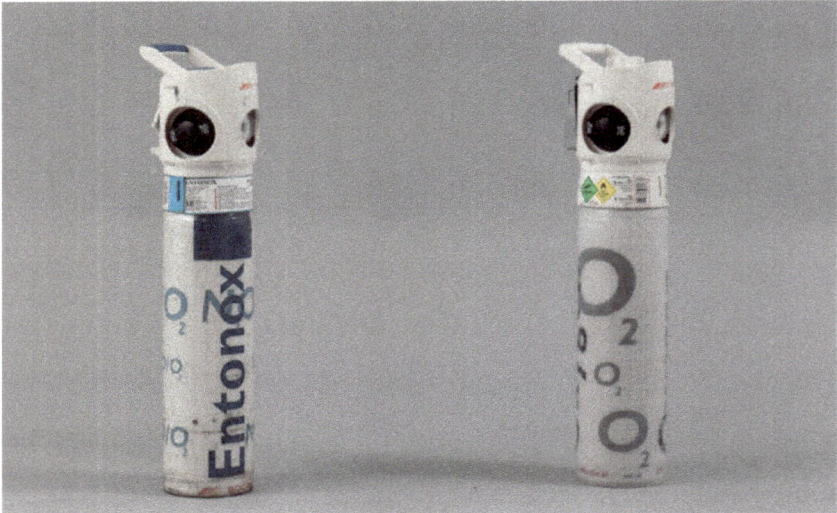

There are two main types of oxygen in use in clinical environments-oxygen and Entonox. The gases are compressed into cylinders, and they have varied sizes.

Oxygen Equipment assembly

The components of an oxygen equipment bag are:

• A therapy mask, a resuscitation mask, tubing, a bag valve mask with a reservoir bag, a regulator, and medical grade oxygen cylinder.

• Lie the cylinder on the floor

• Attach the tube from the non-rebreathe bag or bag valve mask to the oxygen tank

•The cylinder should be turned on

•Flow rate should be set at 15 cylinders when dealing with a critical illness

•Put a mask over the patient's mouth and nose and monitor them.

Disassembly of oxygen cylinder.

•Remove the mask from the patient's face and ensure that the gauge is off until the pressure is at zero.

•The cylinder should be replaced with a new one

Oxygen delivery devices

Non-rebreathe bag-this is used to deliver high concentration oxygen (15 litres of oxygen). The device is made up of a mask and a reservoir bag fitted with a one-way valve. The valve ensures oxygen is inhaled and exhaled air is not returned to the bag.

Simple face Mask-has ports on either side of the mask which allows air to be sucked into the mask.

Classification -Oxygen is a gas.

Action- helps the release of cellular energy.

Indications- hypoxia, ischaemic chest pain, respiratory illnesses, carbon monoxide poisoning, shock, and traumatic injuries

Adverse effects-

- High doses can lead to reduced levels of consciousness.
- High doses of oxygen to a COPD patient can lead to respiratory depression or patients with chronic carbon dioxide retention.
- Oxygen leads to coronary vasoconstriction.

  Contraindications- avoid giving oxygen to patients who have known paraquat poisoning.

Dosage

Low Concentration oxygen

1-4 l/min by nasal cannula

High concentration

10-15 l/min administered through a non-rebreather mask.

Diabetic Emergency medication

MANAGEMENT

Administering Glucose

FAST ACTING CARBOHYDRATE (GLUCOSE)

Oral Glucose

Equipment required- Gloves, Tongue depressor, and PPE.

1. Ensure the patient has no allergies to the medication and if there

is any history of allergic reaction make sure it is documented.

2. Let the patient know what medication you are about to administer and why the medication is necessary.

3. It is important to make sure that the patient is conscious and can swallow.

4. The glucose should be administered buccally between the cheek and the gum.

5. Check that the medication is having the desired effect or note any adverse effects of the medication.

HYPOGLYCAEMIC CHILDREN BETWEEN 0-5 YEARS OLD

Medication	Age of Patient	Route of administration	Dosage	Duration
Glucose	0-5 years	Mouth	5g oral glucose liquid or 20 mL Lift® or 1.5 glucose tablet Or half a tube of 40% oral gel Or 1 teaspoon of sugar dissolved in water	Repeat after 15 minutes if necessary
Glucose	0-5 years	Buccal administration (Conscious but uncooperative children)	5g Or Half a tube of glucose 40% oral gel	Repeat after 15 minutes if necessary

GLUCOGEL (GLUCOSE 40% ORAL GEL)

This is simply sugar which when administered to the patient raises the blood sugar level. The gel is given through the mouth. It is applied to the buccal area of the mouth thereby increasing the rate of absorption to rapidly increase the sugar level. Measure blood sugar level after every dose.

Indications

It should be given to a conscious casualty to avoid the risk of vomit aspiration or choking.

Caution

Where there is a decreased level of consciousness there is a risk of choking. To avoid the risk of aspiration, soak a gauze swab in glucogel and then place it between the patient's lips and gum for easy absorption.

SIDE EFFECTS CONTRAINDICATIONS

None

Repeat the treatment as necessary in a hypoglycaemic patient, but if the treatment fails, resort to glucagon which should be administered intramuscularly, or glucose 10%.

PRESENTATION

One box containing three single-dose plastic tubes of 40% glucose gel (25grams each) sprays depending on the blood pressure.

HYPOGLYCAEMIC CHILDREN BETWEEN THE AGES OF 5-11 YEARS

Medication	Age of the patient	Route of administration	Dosage	Duration
Glucose	5-11	mouth	10g **Or** 40mL Lift® oral glucose liquid **Or** 3 glucose tablets **Or** 1 tube of glucose 40% oral gel **Or** 2 teaspoonfuls of sugar dissolved in water	Repeat after 15 minutes
Glucose	5-11	Buccal administration (Conscious but uncooperative children)	1 tube of glucose 40% oral gel	Repeat 15 minutes if necessary

HYPOGLYCAEMIC CHILDREN BETWEEN 12-17 YEARS

Medication	Age of the patient	Route of administration	Dosage	Duration
Glucose	12-17		15g **Or** 60mL Lift® oral glucose liquid **Or** 4 glucose tablets **Or** 1.5 tube of glucose 40% oral gel **Or** 3 teaspoonfuls of sugar dissolved in water	Repeated every 15 minutes
Glucose	12-17	Buccal	15g	Repeated

	years	administration (Conscious and uncooperative patients)	Or 1.5 tubes of glucose 40% oral gel **Or** 150-200 mL pure fruit juice	after 15 minutes

HYPOGLYCAEMIC ADULTS

Medication	Age of the patient	Route of administration	Dosage	Duration	Body weight
Glucose	Adult	mouth	15-20g **OR** 60-80mL Lift® (formerly known as Glucojuice ®) oral glucose liquid Or 4-5 glucose tablets Or 1.5-2 tubes of glucose 40% oral gel		

			Or 3-4 heaped teaspoonfuls of sugar dissolved in appropriate amounts of water.		
Glucose	Adult	Buccal administration (conscious and uncooperative adults)	15-20g or 1.5-2 tubes of glucose 40% oral gel	Repeated after 15 minutes	

TREATMENT OF HYPOGLYCAEMIC PATIENTS WHERE ORAL ROUTE CAN NOT BE USED

Glucagon injection (GlucoGen®) 1 mg/mL

GLUCAGON

This is a hormone that converts glycogen to glucose in the liver thereby raising the level of sugar in the blood. This medication is injected into a patient whose sugar level is below 4 mmol/L (Hypoglycaemia –low blood sugar) and where a patient is unconscious and low blood sugar is considered the cause of the unconsciousness.

Glucagon injection should be given where giving glucose orally to a patient who is unconscious is not possible or will be ineffective. It is also a better option where administering glucose by IV access is impossible.

CONTRA-INDICATIONS Do not give glucagon by IV injection because it might lead to increased vomiting.

CAUTIONS If the patient has been a recent recipient of glucagon, this may have already caused a low sugar store, so avoid giving the patient glucagon If the patient suffered from hypoglycaemia seizures (seizures triggered by low blood sugar) then avoid giving them glucagon. Glucose 10% IV is a preferred option. It may not be effective in some situations where the low-level sugar has been triggered by excessive alcohol intake.

SIDE EFFECTS Nausea, vomiting, abdominal pain in adults, diarrhoea in children, hypokalaemia, hypotension (low blood pressure) in adults, and, rarely, hypersensitivity reaction.

Medication	Age	Route of administration	Dosage	Duration	Body weight
Glucagon (GlucoGen®)	0-8 years	Intramuscular injection	500 micrograms Or 0.5 mL		Up to 25kg
Glucagon(GlucaGen®)	9-17 years	Intramuscular injection	1mg (1mL)		25kg and over
Glucagon(GlucaGen®)	Adult	Intramuscular injection	1 mg/1mL		

MANAGING AN UNRESPONSIVE HYPOGLYCAEMIA AFTER 10 MINUTES OF TREATMENT WITH GLUCAGON

Medication	Age of the patient	Route of administration	Dosage	Duration	Body weight
Glucose 10% intravenous infusion	child	Intravenous injection through large vein	5mL/kg 500mg/kg		
Glucose 10% intravenous infusion	Adult	Intravenous injection through large vein	120-150 mL	Infused over 15 minutes	
Glucose 20% intravenous infusion	Adult	Intravenous injection through large vein	75-100 mL	Infused over 15 minutes	

SEPSTIC SHOCK

Sepsis shock arises from an exaggerated response of the auto-immune system to infection.

The shock is created by the exaggerated response and not the infection itself.[10] It is not the infection that kills a patient, it is the overreaction of the immune system that leads to fatality.

The systemic inflammatory response creates severe damage to vital organs of the body. The inflammatory reactions create toxins which in turn produce vessel dilation and vascular permeability- (leakage of the blood vessels) and consequently hypovolaemia.

SIGNS AND SYMPTOMS OF SEPSIS

- The patient's body temperature can be either high or low.
- Fast heartbeat and fast breathing
- Slurred speech
- Muscular ache
- Reduced urine output
- Pale, cold clammy skin.
- Signs of recent confusion
- Dizziness,
- feeling faint
- loss of consciousness
- Nausea
- Vomiting

---

[10] Pharmacology for paramedics second edition by Jeffrey S. Guy, P332-333

Management

IV fluids-patients with chronic sepsis require an initial fluid bolus of 30 cc/kg (of actual body weight) within the first 3 hours of resuscitation.

Provision of vasopressor such as noradrenaline

Provision of antibiotics

Measure lactate.

Check urine samples.

Take blood samples to identify infection.

Oxygen-target saturation should be 94-98%; and 88-92 for COPD patients.

Provide fluid therapy- 500ml over 15 hours.

HYPERVENTILATION

This is a rapid deep breathing triggered by panic or anxiety. Excessive breathing caused by panic or anxiety leads to excessive exhalation of carbon dioxide in the blood. Effectively, the patient is breathing more than metabolic requirements[11].

---

[11] Hyperventilation: a practical guide. Medicine 2003, 31(11); 7-8

Signs and symptoms

Dizziness, shortness of breath, dry mouth, weakness, confusion, numbness a tingling sensation around the mouth, palpitations, chest pain, and spasms in the hands and feet.

Treatment

Reassurance, breathing through pursed lips, controls the patient's breathing.

CHRONIC OBSTRUCTIVE PULMONARY DISEASE (COPD)

COPD is a blanket term for a range of respiratory diseases which lead to the obstruction of the airway and are usually progressive and irreversible (Kortext, Page 187) (NICE, 2018). There are two main types of airway diseases that are collectively referred to as Chronic obstructive pulmonary disease. Chronic bronchitis and emphysema-Chronic bronchitis is a daily productive cough that lasts for 3 months of the year and for at least 2 years in a row.

www.nhs.uk>conditions.

Emphysema arises when the air sacs in the lungs become damaged and stretched. COPD stands for chronic pulmonary disease is a condition that affects the lungs and how much oxygen we breathe in and how much carbon dioxide we breathe out. COPD can be caused by a range of factors, particularly pollution, and our work environment but smoking is the most dangerous. The oxygen saturation of those with COPD is often between 88-92% in comparison, the normal oxygen saturation for those without COPD is between 94-99%.

Where the saturation levels for COPD patients exceed 88-92% this can lead to hyperoxia hypercapnia. Hypocapnia is when there is a build-up of carbon dioxide in the body and happens because of hyperoxia. A condition where more oxygen is being used to form carbon dioxide. As a result of COPD, the patient cannot clear out the excess carbon dioxide thereby resulting in the blood becoming acidic. This results in respiratory acidosis and in serious cases can cause death.

It is therefore important that the oxygen saturation levels are checked regularly and this can be achieved by maintaining specific oxygen saturation using the venturi mask and regularly checking oxygen saturation.

SYNCOPE

Fainting is a brief loss of consciousness triggered by a temporary reduction of blood to the brain.

Vasovagal syncope (fainting)- this is a brief loss of consciousness which is normally triggered by a temporary reduction of blood to the brain.

Causes

Fainting occurs when there is a temporary reduction of blood and glucose in the brain due to a drop in cerebral blood pressure.

· It would Usually happen when the person is upright-soon after standing up

· It can happen when sitting down over prolonged periods of inactivity and fainting can also be caused by;

-Drugs

- Dehydration

-Alcohol

-Loss of bodily fluid such as vomiting, bleeding, or diarrhoea.

Signs and symptoms

· Dizziness

· Sweating

· Blurred vision

· Distortion of hearing before collapse

· Might involve jerking which can stop in about twenty seconds

WHEN DOES IT STOP?

When the patient is in a supine position the recovery is rapid. Raise both legs up. Ensure they do not stand up too quickly after recovering. This is to give the blood pressure and heart time to stabilise.

Cardiac Syncope

Cardiac syncope is the result of cardiac dysrhythmia (tachycardia and bradycardia). This is not as common as vasovagal syncope.

It can happen whilst the patient is at rest and can also happen during exercise.

Pre-existing heart disease is a risk factor.

Signs

· Impairment of consciousness lasting over a minute

· Not likely to cause convulsive movements of more than 20 seconds

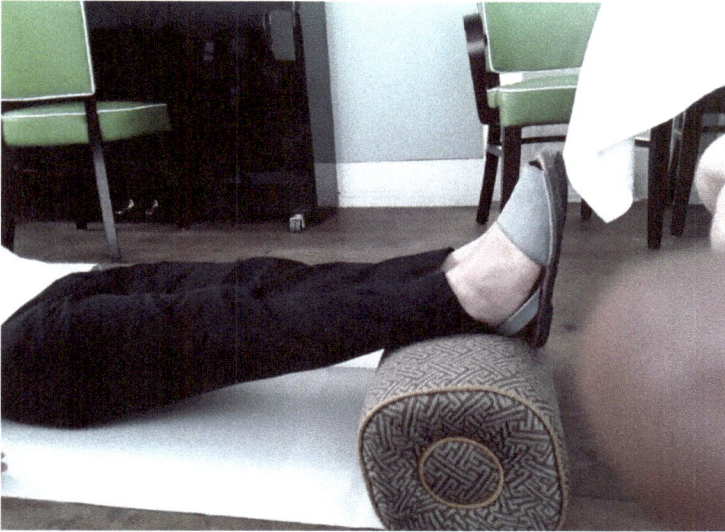

ISBN   978-1-7385061-1-8

Bibliography

CARDIAC ARREST

Acute Coronary syndrome

STEMI

(Vogel B, Claessen BE, Arnold SV, et al. ST-segment elevation myocardial infarction. *Nat Rev Dis Primers*. 2019;5(1):39. doi:10.1038/s41572-019-0090-3)

"Immediate Life Support," Resuscitation Council UK. 5th Edition P17-18, 2021

"ST segment elevation myocardial infarction, the most severe type of heart attack" by Richard.N. Fogoros MD

"Cardiac Biomarkers, Cardiac Enzymes, and heart disease" by Richard N Fogoros, dec 10, 2021

NICE-clinical guidelines 50 Acutely ill adults in hospital London, National Institute for health and clinical Excellence 2007 https://www.nice.org.uk/guidance/cg50

National institute for health and care excellence. Clinical guidelines 167 Myocardial infarction with ST-segment elevation. NICE 2013 www.nice.org.uk/guidance

Nolan JP, J, Smith GB et al Incidence and outcome of in hospital

Cardiac arrest in the United Kingdom National Cardiac arrest audit. Resuscitation 2014, 85:98987-92

Resuscitation council guidelines for safer handling during resuscitation in healthcare settings July 2015 http://www.resus.org.uk/library/publications/publication-guidance-safer-handling

AIRWAY MANAGEMENT

Airway management in cardiopulmonary resuscitation BY Jasmeet Soar and Jerry P. Nolan CURRENT OPINION

SEPSIS

1. Sepsis-crib-cards.pdf

2. Sepsis | Infection prevention and control | Royal College of Nursing (rcn.org.uk) (Royal College of Nursing)

3. Kortex: 240– Ambulance Care Essentials Second Edition by Richard Pilbery and Kriss Lethbridge.

Sepsis-crib-cards.pdf

"The Sepsis Manual" 5th Edition (5th-Edition-manual-080120.pdf (sepsistrust.org))

ASTHMA

Resources:

1. https://www.asthma.org.uk/about/media/facts-and-statistics/
2. https://www.theguardian.com/society/2019/feb/20/revealed-asthmas-deadly-toll-on-young-people-in-the-uk
3. https://www.theguardian.com/environment/2018/jul/04/report-links-childs-asthma-death-to-illegal-levels-of-air-pollution
4. MedicAlert - Medical ID jewellery & services

SEIZURES

Seizures and epilepsy in the acute medical setting: presentation and management (nih.gov)

SYNCOPE

Guidelines for the diagnosis and management of syncope (version 2009)The Task Force for the Diagnosis and Management of Syncope of the European Society of Cardiology (ESC)

Eur Heart J. 2009 Nov; 30(21): 2631–2671.

Published online 2009 Aug 27. doi: 10.1093/eurheartj/ehp298

NATIONAL EARLY WARNING SCORE (NEWS) 2

Standardising the assessment of acute illness in the NHS . Updated Report of a working party Royal College of Physicians. London 2017

SYNCOPE CONTINUED

Vasovagal Syncope | Cedars-Sinai

HYPERVENTILATION

Kashikawa M. Revaluation of paper bag rebreathing for hyperventilation syndrome. International conference and Exhibition on lung Disorder and Therapeutics 2015

Gardner WN-Hyperventilation: A practical Guide, Medicine, 2003, 31(11); 7-8

DNAR

Do not attempt cardiopulmonary resuscitation (DNACPR) decisions - NHS (www.nhs.uk)

ADRT (Advanced decision to refuse treatment)

Advance decision to refuse treatment - Macmillan Cancer Support

CARDIOPULMONARY RESUSCITATION (CPR)

UK resuscitation Council guidelines 2021

CHOKING

About 380 people die from choking every year and most of the deaths are those within the age of 65 years and over

ONS, 2017

Office for National Statistics, 2017. Deaths Registered in England and Wales. Available at: https://www.ons.gov.uk/peoplepopulationandcommunity/birthsde athsandmarriages/deaths/datasets/deathsregisteredinengland

Causes, Prevention, and Treatment of Choking (verywellhealth.com)

Walls, 2012

Walls RM and Murphy MF (eds), 2012. Manual of Emergency Airway

Management. 4th ed. Philadelphia: Wolters Kluwer/Lippincott Williams & Wilkins Health.

What should I do if someone is choking? - NHS (www.nhs.uk)

ASTHMA

Asthma - NHS (www.nhs.uk)

Asthma UK | Homepage

Asthma (who.int)

asthma.pdf (thelancet.com)

CARDIAC ARREST

Acute Coronary syndrome

STEMI

(**Vogel B, Claessen BE, Arnold SV, et al**. ST-segment elevation myocardial infarction. *Nat Rev Dis Primers*. 2019;5(1):39. doi:10.1038/s41572-019-0090-3)

"Immediate Life Support," Resuscitation Council UK. 5th Edition P17-18, 2021

"ST segment elevation myocardial infarction, the most severe type of heart attack" by **Richard .N. Fogoros MD**

"Cardiac Biomarkers, Cardiac enzymes, and heart disease" **by Richard N Fogoros, dec 10, 2021**

NICE-clinical guidelines 50 Acutely ill adults in hospital London, National Institute for health and clinical Excellence 2007 https://www.nice.org.uk/guidance/cg50

National institute for health and Care Excellence. Clinical guidelines 167 Myocardial infarction with ST-segment elevation . NICE 2013 www.nice.org.uk/guidance

Nolan JP, J, Smith GB et al Incidence and outcome of in hospital Cardiac arrest in the United Kingdom National Cardiac arrest audit. Resuscitation 2014, 85:98987-92

Resuscitation council Guidelines for safer handling during resuscitation in healthcare settings July 2015 http://www.resus.org.uk/library/publications/publication-guidance-safer-handling

AIRWAY MANAGEMENT

Airway management in cardiopulmonary resuscitation **BY Jasmeet Soara and Jerry P. Nolanb** CURRENT OPINION

NATIONAL EARLY WARNING SCORE (NEWS) 2

Standardising the assessment of acute illness in the NHS. Updated Report of a working party Royal College of Physicians. London 201

DNAR

Do not attempt cardiopulmonary resuscitation (DNACPR) decisions - NHS (www.nhs.uk)

ADRT Advanced decision to refuse treatment.

Advance decision to refuse treatment - Macmillan Cancer Support

CARDIOPULMONARY RESUSCITATION (CPR)

UK resuscitation Council guidelines 2021

CHOKING

About 380 people die from choking every year and most of the deaths are those within the age of 65 years and over

ONS, 2017

Office for National Statistics, 2017. Deaths Registered in England and Wales. Available at:
https://www.ons.gov.uk/peoplepopulationandcommunity/birthsde athsandmarriages/deaths/datasets/deathsregisteredinengland

Causes, Prevention, and Treatment of Choking (verywellhealth.com)

Walls, 2012

Walls RM and Murphy MF (eds), 2012. Manual of Emergency Airway Management. 4th ed. Philadelphia: Wolters Kluwer/Lippincott Williams & Wilkins Health.

What should I do if someone is choking? - NHS (www.nhs.uk)

www.ingramcontent.com/pod-product-compliance
Lightning Source LLC
Chambersburg PA
CBHW051246020426
42333CB00025B/3076